I Never Told Anyone

I NEVER TOLD ANYONE

Writings by Women Survivors of Child Sexual Abuse

edited by

Ellen Bass and Louise Thornton

with

Jude Brister, Grace Hammond,
Jean Huntley, and Vicki Lamb

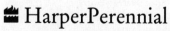 HarperPerennial

A Division of HarperCollins*Publishers*

Grateful acknowledgment is made to the following publishers and authors for permission to reprint:

Excerpt from *I Know Why the Caged Bird Sings*, by Maya Angelou. Copyright © 1969 by Maya Angelou. Reprinted by permission of Random House, Inc.

Excerpt from *Lady Sings the Blues* by Billie Holiday with William F. Dufty. Copyright © 1956 by Eleanora Fagan and William F. Dufty. Reprinted by permission of Doubleday & Co., Inc.

Excerpt from *Flying*, by Kate Millett. Copyright © 1974 by Kate Millett. Reprinted by permission of Alfred A. Knopf, Inc., and the author.

"First Time: 1950" copyright © 1980 by Honor Moore. Reprinted by permission of the author.

Other selections included in this anthology are printed here by arrangement with the individual authors. Previous publication information is included in the author's biography which precedes each piece.

A hardcover edition of this book was published in 1983 by Harper & Row, Publishers.

First Harper Colophon edition published 1983. First HarperPerennial edition published 1991.

Library of Congress Cataloging-in-Publication Data

I never told anyone: writings by women survivors of child sexual abuse/edited by Ellen
   Bass, Louise Thornton; with Jude Brister . . . [et al.].
      p.   cm.
   Includes bibliographical references.
      ISBN 0-06-096573-8 (pbk.)
      1. Adult child sexual abuse victims—United States—Biography.   2. Sexually
   abused children—United States—Biography.   3. Abused women—United States—
   Biography.   I. Bass, Ellen.   II. Thornton, Louise.   III. Brister, Jude.
   HQ72.U53I14 1991   90-55489
   362.7′6—dc20

---

91 92 93 94 95 AG/MB 10 9 8 7 6 5 4 3 2

To the children

CONTENTS

Contents   7

NOTE TO THE NEW PAPERBACK EDITION

For this new edition of *I Never Told Anyone: Writings By Women Survivors of Child Sexual Abuse,* none of the original stories has been changed. The biographies of the contributors also remain the same, except for the addition of recent publications. However, the resources have been entirely redone and reflect the increase of supportive services and useful, inspiring books. There is also the addition of an afterword in which Ellen Bass reflects on the gains that have been achieved in the last decade of survivors' healing from child sexual abuse, as well as the essential work still to be done.

Acknowledgments

We would like to thank all of the women who sent manuscripts to us. All of these writings were intrinsic to the creation of this anthology whether or not they were included. While we received many more writings than we could use because of space limitations, we felt privileged to be able to read each one. Knowing there were so many who had been sexually abused as children deepened our commitment to compiling this book. We are immensely grateful to all those who so courageously shared their lives with us and wish them strength and peace.

We would also like to thank Bill Minkner, Vee Duvall, and Parents United for their cooperation and experience; Ray Gwyn Smith, Jill Ginghofer, Mariah Burton Nelson, and Lyle Fleming for reading and responding to the manuscript: Santa Cruz Women Against Rape for their donation and use of their library; and Sally Cooper for her assistance.

We especially thank Lucy Diggs for endless typing, patience, and advice.

Finally, we thank our families and friends for their support and understanding during the four years we worked on this book.

FOREWORD
Florence Rush

I never told anyone: Why is it that children who have been molested, sexually abused, or even raped rarely or never tell? They never tell for the same reason that anyone who has been helplessly shamed and humiliated, and who is without protection or validation of personal integrity, prefers silence. Like the woman who has been raped, the violated child may not be believed (she fantasized or made up the story), her injury may be minimized (there's no harm done, so let's forget the whole thing), and she may even be held accountable for the crime (the kid really asked for it).

A growing child gains self-esteem and confidence from the value placed upon her by adults whom she trusts and upon whom she must depend. The sexually exploited child, however, rarely elicits a reaction necessary to promote a positive identity. Unsupported in her right to be protected, to be angry, or to express justified indignation, she feels she deserves no more than to be sexually used. To expose an incident is to expose her own insignificance. To tell anyone is to be disgraced in her own eyes and the eyes of others. The child victim has no recourse but to bury, hide, and try to forget the experience. But the humiliation will not go away. It festers, poisons and undermines her being. When the offense remains hidden, unanswered and unchallenged, the sexuality, the very biology of the offended child, becomes her shame.

This destructive syndrome did not arise in a vacuum. It stems from age-old traditions and customs that are written in history, religion, law, and in today's powerful and influential media. In the beginning of our Western civilization, the female, along with a house, ox, and ass, was a man's property. Specifically, she was a sexual property whose only destiny was to provide progeny and pleasure, and her value was determined by the compensation she could bring as either a breeder or prostitute. This is the ignominious heritage we have bequeathed to our female children.

The sexual abuse of little girls is predicated upon their presumed inferiority. A little girl can be used sexually because she is property, or because she is biologically imperfect, or because she is an enticing, sexy temptress. Simultaneously defined and degraded by her sexuality, she is constrained within a foolproof system of emotional blackmail. If she is violated, the culturally imposed concept of her sexuality renders her culpable. Any attempt on the part of the child to expose her violator also exposes her own alleged inferiority and sexual motives and shames her rather than the offender. Concealment is her only alternative.

But we, as women, are beginning to refute our training that we are inferior, and will no longer be blackmailed or constrained. We are now pointing a finger at our abusers. They are the guilty ones. The women within these pages, despite the pitfalls, snares, and risks, are stronger, prouder, and feel better about themselves because at last they have the courage to tell their stories. The lesson to be learned from this testimony is to believe in and to protect the integrity of our children and to break the silence that endangers them.

PREFACE
Louise Thornton

This collection of women's voices speaks out about what is seldom said, seldom told, seldom acknowledged—the sexual violation of children. It is about the silence of nights spent holding in screams, holding back tears, holding in one's very self. And it is about the stillness of days when all of a young girl's resources are used up in keeping the secret from everyone, sometimes even herself. The women in this anthology are breaking this silence. Whether by whispers or cries or shouts or screams, they will continue to shatter it with the power of their own voices, their own words.

This anthology grew out of a women's writing workshop led by Ellen Bass. One winter afternoon in Santa Cruz, California, a group including myself sat listening to a story Jude Brister was reading. In this story, "The Window's Netting," a girl of eleven is raped by her father. When the story ended, we sat quietly, the only sound that of rain drumming against the windows. After a while someone asked, "Did that really happen?" "Yes," Jude answered. "My God!" someone else said.

As we discussed the story, Ellen told us that she had heard many similar stories or poems in her workshops. She felt that child sexual abuse must be fairly common and said that for some time she had wanted to put together a collection of writings about the experience. As the class ended, Jude Brister, Grace Hammond, Jean Huntley, Vicki Lamb, and I approached Ellen about editing the anthology with her.

We asked ourselves two questions as we began working on the book: What kinds of writings did we want to include, and why did we want to edit such a book? As we talked we realized that we were looking for poems and stories written by those who had personally experienced child sexual abuse in any of its manifestations. This abuse happens anytime an adult or near-adult takes away the child's right to exclusive ownership of her body. It is accomplished either by manipulation of the child's feelings or by force. It ranges from making her feel that daddy will be miserable unless he can fondle her to brutal sexual assault. It includes the sliding of a dressmaker's hand into a child's panties even as her mother is talking to a nearby clerk, or prolonged, full-mouth kissing by a neighbor the child has known all her life. In all of these instances, the child has lost power over her body, over her sexuality, over her very self.

While this is a book about the experiences of women, we are aware that boys as well as girls are sexually abused. Just recently a well-known poet, Rod McKuen, began to speak openly of how he was molested as a child. Shortly after we began working on this book, Shel Horowitz sent us a poem he had written about being raped by an older male when he was small. In an accompanying letter, he said, "Growing up as a boy I was totally innocent of such things as rape. My parents had always given us general warnings about staying away from strangers, but I avoided the kind of indoctrination my sisters were given. I was thus completely unprepared for what happened and internalized a great deal of guilt. I knew it was wrong, but felt somehow it was my own fault." Shel also told us that several of his male friends were molested as children and that he believed male-male rape to be far more common than most people realize.

We are grateful to Shel for sharing his feelings with us and hope that the experiences of men who have been sexually abused as children will also be told.

The process of compiling this anthology began with requesting writings from women we knew personally who had survived child sexual abuse. We then placed notices in literary and feminist newsletters asking for stories and poems written by other survivors. We hoped to find clear, strong, distilled writing, "life refined," as Gwendolyn Brooks says about her poetry. We hoped to find writers who would take an experience as horrendous as being sexually abused as a child and, like Picasso with the bombing of Guernica, turn it into a work of art.

As we began to receive such manuscripts, we came to understand exactly why we were putting together the anthology: to help give the sexually abused child a voice. She had been studied, evaluated, reevaluated, and compiled into numerous statistics and case studies. But had this child ever spoken for herself?

"I told no one," one of our contributors wrote us. "My primary response was silence."

Another wrote, "I couldn't tell anyone about my grandfather molesting me when I was eight. My grandmother was a particularly wonderful and loving woman. I felt that if I told her or anyone I would be destroying her marriage as well as destroying my family."

One woman spoke of telling her first boyfriend in the vaguest terms about a prolonged incestuous relationship with her father. "I was too filled with shame, guilt, and embarrassment to give him a detailed account," she explained. "I thought if I told him too much he might think I was 'sick.' "

Rarely does the child tell. Not only has her physical self been violated; she feels that her integrity has been lost. This is the most difficult part to speak about openly, for how does a child say that she no longer feels good about herself, that she feels only an inner dissolution?

"Powerlessness and masochism still feel right," one contributor stated. "This powerlessness has drained me many times of my dignity as a human being. I become a thing."

Jill Morgan, who was sexually abused throughout childhood, wrote, "I have attempted suicide more times than I care to count, and only my rock-bound determination to survive has kept me going."

Blanche Woodbury voiced the other side of this lack of self-esteem: "I still seek 'worldly success' to prove I am worthy of being alive ... A's in school, publication of my writing ... always the search for redemption."

This assumption of guilt and the ensuing shame is perhaps the primary reason why the sexually abused child does not tell. A second reason is the child's belief that her word alone will very likely not be honored. Phyllis Koestenbaum, who was molested as a child at a football game, wanted desperately to tell her mother about the abuse, but could not. "Did I think she'd accuse me," she asks herself, "or maybe deny the reality of what happened? Say it couldn't have happened as she denied other things I told her?"

Recently I talked to a very confused and anxious young woman who was abused by her father for six years during her childhood. "Did you ever receive any help in dealing with the abuse?" I asked her. "Oh," she answered, "I went to a psychiatrist when I was fourteen. My mother took me. But he said I had an overactive imagination. I made up the whole thing! So my mother told me to just forget about it."

Several contributors to this anthology wrote me that they received a similar response when they told a psychiatrist about their own experiences. I do not want to imply that all professional counselors respond in such a manner; many of our contributors attributed their healing in part to the skilled and compassionate help of therapists, particularly feminist therapists. Yet there exists the tendency to betray the abused child a second time by blaming her "overactive imagination" rather than confronting the fact that daddy, uncle, or grandpa is indeed capable of molesting a child. (See the Introduction and the discussion of Freud for elaboration on the background of this tendency.)

Or the child does not tell because she is made to feel that she was an accomplice, that she enjoys being sexually abused even though she says clearly that she does not. In some instances the child's body may respond to the sexual stimulation even as her consciousness is horrified. In an article on incest published in *City on a Hill* (June 5, 1980), Jeanne Modesitt wrote, "One evening after my father had fondled me for about an hour, my body involuntarily climaxed. I had never experienced orgasm before. I was frightened and disgusted as I looked up at my father and saw his triumphant smile. I felt as if my body had betrayed me. I began to hate myself."

Because she does not know that her body can respond without her consent, or even that it can respond in such a way at all, the abused child feels that she must have wanted the abuse, must have asked for it in some way. It is this betrayal of herself by her body that she sometimes finds the hardest to forgive. And again, she does not tell; she fears that anyone she tells would surely blame her as much as she blames herself.

Our primary hope for this anthology is that the sexually abused child will come to understand that she can tell. In this telling she can reclaim her innocence. She *is* innocent. She has *always* been innocent. Both the burden of the crime and the crime itself are lifted from her shoulders. She can tell.

The women in this anthology are telling despite the confusion of feelings some of them are still experiencing. From the beginning, some contributors have made it very clear that the only way they could even consider having their stories or poems published was to use a pseudonym. Other contributors, more than half, were equally clear that they wanted to use their legal names to identify themselves and their experiences. While they often changed the names of anyone identifiable within the writing, this was only because of the law regarding invasion of privacy. As we compiled the anthology, we respected the needs of both those women who wanted to use their own names and those who needed to protect themselves or their families through using a pseudonym. Again and again we were wrenched by the deepening realization that the pressure against telling, of going against thousands of years of keeping child sexual abuse hidden and therefore ongoing, was still almost overwhelming.

Yet the women in this anthology have told, are telling, will tell. Their courage and strength have nurtured us. Recently I received a letter from Jill Morgan expressing concern about the biography I had written of her. "It echoes what I have told you over these three years, yet the tone vaguely alarms me." She then explained what she felt was missing: her strength in surviving her childhood.

She continued: "A close personal friend (male) has asked me repeatedly, 'Why do you have to rehash it? It happened. It's over. Now forget it and go on.' Only by owning myself and my past, by affirming and confirming my innocence in the whole, sordid drama can I rest and feel comfortable with myself.

"If my survival is to be meaningful at all to me, it must be because it gave me the strength to fight, the will to survive and the empathy to reach out to other women. I am (now) a strong, capable, and loving woman partly because of the trauma and despair of the past. Only when you push yourself (or are pushed) to the very limits can you test the strength of your endurance and power."

I feel as if I know Jill intimately even though we have never met. Because she says, "I am now a strong, capable, loving woman," I believe I can also say it about myself. She has said it for me and for all women whether we have survived child sexual abuse or other forms of despair. We as women are strong and vital. As Lynn Swenson, another contributor, says, "I believe not only in my ability to survive, but to flourish."

This anthology is divided into several sections. It begins with a foreword by Florence Rush, who wrote *The Best Kept Secret,* a book chronicling the historical and sociological customs that have sanctioned child sexual abuse for thousands of years. In the Introduction, Ellen Bass places child sexual abuse in a broad social context, discussing its age-old history and its place in our present culture, which continues to allow such abuse. Speaking to all women, and their children, she talks about the psychology of abusers; the role of advertising and the media; the overwhelming pervasiveness of child sexual abuse and the various explanations and justifications for it; and she speaks of her fears for her own young daughter and her small triumphs in finding ways to protect her and teach her to protect herself.

In the body of the book, we have grouped the writings into four categories. Those telling of child sexual abuse by fathers are the first of these. Because of the unique character of this type of abuse in terms of betrayal and devastation, we felt these pieces needed to be set apart from the others. The second group includes writings about sexual abuse by relatives: grandparents, stepfathers, uncles, brothers—all people whom the child has every right to believe she can trust. The third group tells of sexual abuse by friends and acquaintances: baby-sitters, priests, pastors, house painters, neighbors, day-care workers. The last category tells of sexual abuse by someone we have perhaps been the most conditioned to expect it from: the stranger. However, the molesters written about in this section seldom fit the "dirty old man" stereotype. One molester is a soldier, one the manager of a shoe store, another a well-dressed vacationer at a summer resort.

As a child, one of our editors came upon someone she loved very much being abused by a respected family friend. In writing about this incident, she realized that she, too, had been molested at an early age. "It comes back to me," she wrote, "my 'friendly' uncle picking me up, putting his hands in my pants, feeling my vulva, stroking a few times, holding me tight." She continued: "It doesn't matter if you live in the city or in the country, if your family is together or apart, if you're black or white, rich or poor; any child is vulnerable."

Because of this vulnerability, we have also included a comprehensive, state-by-state listing of treatment and prevention programs at the end of the book. If you are a parent or teacher who wants to teach children about child sexual abuse and how to protect themselves, please turn to this section. If you have been or are now involved in child sexual abuse, you may also want to learn of the nearest support group. Grace Hammond describes a particularly exciting program for children called Safe, Strong and Free. Vicki Lamb talks about her work with Parents United programs, which are designed for both the abused and those who have been the abusers. To complete the resource information, we have included a selected list of recommended reading and audiovisual materials for both adults and children.

As you begin to read this anthology, you may at times find yourself overwhelmed with grief and rage. Please allow these feelings. We are human, sentient beings. We feel in order to remain healthy and sane. If we do not feel, we become numb or callous, and a vital part of us dies. Once you feel the initial horror of those who have written about this traumatic aspect of their childhoods and then gradually integrate it into yourself, you will also be able to experience with them their final victory of self-acceptance and wholeness.

We sincerely hope that this anthology will help prevent further child sexual abuse. Someone who is molesting a child can be helped through counseling to obtain a healed, positive self-image. Adults who are filled with self-contempt and a sense of powerlessness vent these feelings on the bodies of vulnerable children. Adults who love and value themselves also love and value children and allow them inalienable rights to their own bodies. Children, in turn, can be taught that their bodies are theirs, that they have a right to them above any other person.

The women in these pages have transformed themselves, like phoenixes rising from the ashes, through their own words. Ideally this anthology will unlock the power of the spoken or written word for the thousands of additional women who never told anyone.

INTRODUCTION:

In the Truth Itself, There Is Healing

Ellen Bass

Years ago, in my writing workshop, a woman wrote of her experience: a small child, asleep in her bed, her father's whispers, his hands between her legs, the pain, confusion, fear, blurred in sleep. In waking, his penis in her mouth, forced against her throat, the gagging, the vomit, the repetition through childhood, into adolescence—a cycle of rape, shame, and unshared, unshareable torment. This woman read her words aloud. Slowly and with great effort, with perseverance, with willingness to face the pain, the rage, the disgust—with courage, with tears, with integrity, with hunger for survival and for a meaningful, nurturing life, she spoke the words, she mourned her past, she celebrated her survival, her strength.

Another woman, farther back, a slight wisp of a girl-woman, woman-child, not yet twenty. She wanted to write—her words on scraps of paper, half-sheets, envelopes. She brought them to me tucked between pages of a notebook, stuffed into her purse. Apologizing, she fumbled through papers, searched for the page, and finally, showed me her writing. Her meanings were hidden: She used words to veil, to obscure. She wanted to write her story, but the task was unfathomable. She could not face what had happened to her—her guilt, her fury, her memory of helplessness, isolation. But she did not give up. She wrote. She began typing fragments; she used full sheets of paper; she constructed whole paragraphs. She sought her mother and talked with her. She was slow and relentless. She married, bore a daughter, cut funny card-board shapes to make her a mobile, and nursed her in the pre-dawn lightening of the sky. And between cooking, working, driving, cleaning, feeding the baby, loving, and sleeping, she wrote. She stayed up late to write; she wrote while the baby napped. She told her story. She published it in a college literary journal—and won a prize. This woman is Maggie Hoyal and her story, "These Are the Things I Remember," is included here.

These women—and more—women whose courage gives me courage, whose lives are a testament to the strength and beauty of women—our rugged tenacity; our unwillingness, in the midst of widespread, smothering violence and a history of atrocities, to give up, give in, die—these women inspired me to collect these stories. In the process of writing, of saying what has not been said, of giving voice to the unnameable, we claim our experience. We are brave. We are no longer victims. We show what we have endured. We look at this reality in order to destroy it.

The Abuse Is Extensive

The sexual abuse of children spans all races, economic classes, and ethnic groups. Even babies are its victims—hospitals treat three-month-old infants for venereal disease of the throat. Sexually abused children are no more precocious, pretty, or sexually curious than other children. They do not ask for it. They do not want it. Like rape of women, the rape and molestation of children are most basically acts of violation, power, and domination.

Parents United, a self-help support group for people who have been involved with child molestation, estimates that one out of four girls and one out of seven boys will be sexually abused. Other studies find the ratio of girls to be higher, closer to ten girls for each boy. The sex of the molester, however, is consistent from study to study. At least 97 percent of child molesters and rapists are men; 75 percent are family members, men well known to the child.[1] These are statistics. Because the majority of abuses are not reported, exact figures are impossible to obtain. The true numbers may be greater. But even these show clearly that the sexual abuse of children is common; that the abusers are men—not exceptional, but average; that the victims are mostly girls—not exceptional, but ordinary. This is violence by men against children, and although there can be individual explanations, individual resolution, and though there is always individual pain, individual wounding, scarring, the issue is not an individual issue but a societal one. We live in a society where men are encouraged to do violence to women and children, subtly and overtly.

Professionals Advocate the Sexual Use of Children

Many of our institutions seek to eradicate all sense of guilt, all standards of decency, all respect for another's bodily integrity. When Freud was confronted with frequent accounts of sexual assault by fathers against daughters in his psychiatric practice, he felt he had discovered a major cause of hysteria. But as the enormity of this indictment against fathers became apparent to him, and as he "inferred from the existence of some hysterical features in his brother and several sisters that even his father had been thus incriminated," he revised his opinion and decided that women had fantasized these rapes.[2]

Today psychologists, psychiatrists, anthropologists, and researchers no longer deny the reality of sex between adults and

1. For sources on the scope of child sexual abuse, see *Conspiracy of Silence: The Trauma of Incest* by Sandra Butler (New York: Bantam, 1978), *Against Our Will: Men, Women and Rape* by Susan Brownmiller (New York: Bantam, 1975), and *The Best Kept Secret: Sexual Abuse of Children* by Florence Rush (Englewood Cliffs, N.J.: Prentice-Hall, 1980). All of these cite a variety of studies to which you can refer for more complete statistics.

2. Ernest Jones, *The Life and Work of Sigmund Freud* (New York: Basic Books, 1961), p. 211. Quoted by Florence Rush in *The Best Kept Secret* (Englewood Cliffs, N.J.: Prentice-Hall, 1980), p. 91. See Rush's entire chapter, "A Freudian Cover-Up."

children. Instead, a growing number rename it, calling it a "sexual encounter," "sexual experience," or "sexual relationship," and give their approval.

John Money of The Johns Hopkins University says, "A childhood sexual experience, such as being the partner of a relative or of an older person, need not necessarily affect the child adversely."[3]

Wardell Pomeroy, coauthor of the Kinsey report, says, "it is time to admit that incest need not be a perversion or a symptom of mental illness. Incest between ... children and adults ... can sometimes be beneficial."[4]

Yehudi Cohen, an anthropologist at Rutgers University, writes, "The incest taboo may indeed be obsolete."[5]

Larry Constantine, an assistant clinical professor of psychiatry at Tufts University, says, "Children have the right to express themselves sexually, even with members of their own family."[6]

And Seymour Parker, an anthropologist from the University of Utah, writes in a paper entitled "The Waning of the Incest Taboo," "It is questionable if the costs [of the incest taboo] in guilt and uneasy distancing between intimates are necessary or desirable. What are the benefits of linking a mist of discomfort to the spontaneous warmth of the affectionate kiss and touch between family members?"[7]

These kinds of attitudes can distort the authentic needs of the abused child and ignore the anguish documented here. There can be no equality of power, understanding, or freedom in sex between adults and children. Children are dependent upon adults:

3. Quoted in "Attacking the Last Taboo," *Time* magazine, April 14, 1980, p. 72.
4. Ibid.
5. Yehudi Cohen, "The Disappearance of the Incest Taboo," *Human Nature,* July 1978, p. 78.
6. "Attacking the Last Taboo."
7. Quoted in "Attacking the Last Taboo" and Benjamin DeMott, "The Pro-Incest Lobby," *Psychology Today,* March 1980, p. 12.

first, for their survival; then for affection, attention, and an under-standing of what the world in which they live is all about.

Though there may be no physical force involved, every time a child is sexually used by a man, there is coercion. A child submits to sex with a man for many reasons: She is afraid to hurt the man's feelings; she wants and needs affection and this is the only form in which it's being offered; she is afraid that if she resists, the man will hurt her or someone else; she is afraid that if she resists, the man will say she started it and get her in trouble; she is taken by surprise and has no idea what to do; the man tells her it's okay, the man says he's teaching her, the man says everybody does it; she has been taught to obey adults; she thinks she has no choice.

Children trust the adults in their lives, even when the adults are untrustworthy, because they have no choice. When that trust is betrayed, they learn the world is not dependable.

By actions as well as by words, adults teach children what to fear, what to trust, what is good, bad, shameful, safe, possible. Children either accept our definitions or, if their experience is radically different (as it is for children who are molested), they are thrown into conflict, confusion, insecurity, and anguish.

When a man sexually uses a child, he is giving that child a strong message about her world: He is telling her that she is important because of her sexuality, that men want sex from girls, and that relationships are insufficient without sex. He is telling her that she can use her sexuality as a way to get the attention and affection she genuinely needs, that sex is a tool. When he tells her not to tell, she learns there is something about sex that is shameful and bad; and that she, because she is a part of it, is shameful and bad; and that he, because he is a part of it, is shame-ful and bad. She learns that the world is full of sex and is shameful and bad and not to be trusted, that even those entrusted with her care will betray her; that she will betray herself.

Although sometimes a child is able to say no, most children are not able to say no even when they desperately want to. Fortunately, programs are being developed to teach children how to refuse sexual advances, unwanted touching, and other invasions of their persons,[8] but even though these programs are immensely valuable, there is no way to equalize the basic inequality of power, understanding, or freedom between a child and an adult.

A Good Excuse

After publishing an excerpt from this book in *Matrix*, the Santa Cruz women's news magazine, I received a call from a local self-defined psychologist and sex researcher who was disturbed by my "indictments" of men such as John Money and Larry Constantine. He told me he believed that children had sexual feelings and should be permitted to express them, even with adults. Perhaps we could meet and talk further, he suggested. I wanted to hang up, but I felt I should take advantage of this opportunity to talk to him. Working on this anthology, the question has come up again and again: Why? Why do men feel they have the right to use children sexually? Although I understand something of the tradition of our society that sanctions the abuse of women and children for men's pleasure or convenience, still there is a level of not understanding, of never being able to understand *why*. And *how*. How does a man split himself so thoroughly that he convinces himself it is acceptable, even *good*, to use children sexually? We arranged a meeting.

---

8. For example, the Child Assault Prevention Project of Women Against Rape, Columbus, Ohio, has developed an excellent program that they present in elementary schools for teachers, parents, and children. Their pioneering work in teaching children ways to become "safe, strong, and free" is a hopeful model that could—and should—be extended across the country.

A number of publications, including some of those listed in the bibliography, include guidelines for parents and other adults to help children protect themselves.

Parents United groups in many cities also speak in schools, teaching children that they have a right to protect themselves from sexual abuse and offering help.

Louise Thornton and I talked with him for two hours. The meeting was frustrating and deeply disturbing. As I have experienced before with men who do not want to confront their abuse of women and children, our questions were often not directly answered, answers contradicted each other, and—what was most revealing to me—when we pointed out that his condescension and hatred for women and girls was apparent even in his language (for example, he referred to girls as "prick teasers"), he dismissed it as an issue of semantics.

The sexual abuse of children is too widespread to put much emphasis on the childhood or background of individual molesters as being the cause of later behavior. Yet when this man recounted his background, I found myself saying, silently, *Of course.* He was, he said, the by-product of his parents' last attempt at reconciliation. By the time he was born, his father was gone and his mother, not wanting, he said, a male child, took his older sister and left the state, abandoning him on the back porch. After hospitalization for pneumonia, he was placed in the home of two women who, he said, at times disciplined him abusively but also showed him love, allowing his "feminine" side and his softness. They taught him sewing, embroidery, cooking. His childhood, he said, was mostly happy.

His adolescence was guilt-ridden in terms of sexual feelings. The influence of the church and society combined to make him feel guilty for wanting to kiss a girl or hold her hand. "I don't have many resentments," he told us, "but I certainly do resent that in the marvelous flush of youth and love and tenderness, that I was disallowed to express my feelings by society."

He became a minister and he married a woman who, he told us, was closed off from her sexuality. "I became a sex therapist trying to figure her out," he said. Now he has pieced together that she must have been sexually abused as a very young child. They have since separated. He also told us, "I got her orgasmic in eighteen months."

When I asked, "*You* got *her* orgasmic? Didn't you do it together?" he said, "No. I don't think I ever reached her mind."

And I never reached his. He could not understand why I found his language—"I got her orgasmic"—so offensive. Yet this small phrase reflects a well of disrespect, a vision of woman as object, to be "reached," "figured out," "got orgasmic." There is no joining in partnership, no shared desire, no equality. Just as in sex between an adult and a child, there is no equality.

He went on to describe the René Guyon Society, of which he is a member. This group, as he explained it, advocates sex between children and adults within prescribed circumstances called "ethics." Children are "free" to sexually explore adults; the adults are not to initiate or further the exploration. As an example, he recounted his own experience at a rural commune where a seven-year-old girl fondled his penis, on her own initiative, he said, until it was erect. He didn't want to tell her to stop, he said, because he didn't want to give her the feeling she was doing something wrong.

What he could not hear from us, what he did not want to hear because it would have cut off his access to the bodies of children, is that we deceive ourselves—and the children—gravely in pretending that their actions are autonomous, unrelated to what they sense we want of them. Children need our approval, our affirmation, so deeply that (when they are not breaking free) they reflect whom we want them to be. Growing up in a society that emphasizes sex, and in a subculture that outlines "acceptable" sexual behavior for children with adults, in which the adults are desirous of "playing with" (to use his language) children and being sexually played with, many children—most children, perhaps—will act out this behavior. But it is not they who initiate. The adults who set up this code are the initiators. The children follow their expectations.

I am mother to a four-year-old daughter, Sara. When she was a toddler and her father or I were undressed, drying off from a shower or putting our clothes on in the morning, she would sometimes comment on our genitals, saying "vagina" and patting my vagina, or "penis" and touching her father's penis. We would say, "Yes, that's my vagina," or "Yes, that's my penis," let her pat for a moment, and continue drying or dressing. She would perhaps comment that our dog, Sunshine, has a penis, too, or that she has a vagina, too, or that her teddy bear has a penis, in which case I might remind her that it looks like a penis but it's meant to be a tail. I consider this healthy. She is curious about the world, and genitals are a part of it. At that point they held no more fascination for her than bees, large trucks, or swings—less fascination than swings. It would not have been healthy for me to lie back, spread my legs, and "allow" her to fondle my vagina, pretending to myself that she was the initiator. That would have been a lie. It would have been a violation of her even if I never touched her, as this man assured us repeatedly he never touched children.

Just before the interview was to end, however, he went on to say that once a child was "physically mature"—adolescent—she or he "may choose" a lover/teacher to initiate her or him. He himself had initiated two thirteen-year-old girls, one having lived with him for two months. All this, he explained, was approved by the girls' parents beforehand.

He told this in careful speech, one hand hovering about his mouth, often shielding it, emphasizing that "I have to be extraordinarily cautious about what I say and where I say it. I'd get crucified," he added, "and I'm not a martyr."

A few days after this meeting, friends came to visit with a thirteen-year-old daughter. She had just been accepted as a cheerleader and was eager to show us the cheers she had learned. The routines were implicitly sexual and explicitly violent:

"Hit 'em again, hit 'em again. Harder, harder."

"We're going all the way. We're busting up okay."

"We are vicious, malicious, and will put you to the test."

"Get your butt and spin around."

The accompanying movements were meant to be provocative. She performed them with a mixture of enthusiasm and embarrassment. Our daughter, Sara, loved watching her jumps, kicks, and clapping hands. She called, "More tricks! More tricks!" jumping and clapping herself. The new cheerleader did "tricks." I was struck with the renewed knowledge of how young a thirteen-year-old girl is—her energy was closer to Sara's than to ours. And I was again made aware of how our society, even our schools, teach children to act out provocative behavior[9]—behavior that irresponsible men then take as license to use girls sexually.

Thirteen is the age of initiation in the René Guyon Society. Thirteen is the age at which this man calls girls "prick teasers" if they kiss or fondle and don't come through with intercourse. This is the age at which he—and the René Guyon Society—"allow" (which means encourage) children to enter into sexual relationships with adults, as though sex were primarily a skill, an area of life in which one is taught to be competent. This is the age at which he advocates that parents, having provided their daughters with information about birth control much earlier, now provide the birth control itself. They give the child a choice, of course, of which method to use, but they never face the fact that there is *no* birth control that is both safe to the girl's health and totally reliable. They never face the possibility of pregnancy—the life-and-death choice of abortion that is anguishing even for many adult women, unfair and cruel to put in the hands of a child.

What emerged was the portrait of a man who had not experienced the joy of his own sexual awakening, whose first "marvel-

---

9. At one local high school, cheerleaders wear ultrashort skirts, black lace tights, and a single garter.

ous flush of . . . love and tenderness" was called "dirty" and subsequently suppressed. No one will deny the pain of all such suppressions of the body and the spirit. But rather than encouraging young people to express their sexuality together, with appropriate limits, with open, informed, and caring discussion, and with the affirmation that our sexual feelings are a beautiful expression of the life force, of renewal and of loving, this man has bought into a system of "ethics" that makes it acceptable for him to be lovers with the thirteen-year-old girls he was not permitted to kiss or hold hands with or fondle forty years ago.

Louise and I left the interview feeling we had said little of what we had really wanted to say and that very little of that had permeated his construct of how he wanted sex to be. I felt frustrated and deeply tired, grateful only that the meeting was over. Although I was unable to express my opinions in a satisfying way, someone else—a young person, appropriately—did it for me. When Louise was telling her husband about this man's views on adolescent initiation and the lover/teacher relationship, her fifteen-year-old son was listening. He remarked succinctly, "It sounds like a good excuse."

The History: Ownership and Desecration

People are becoming alarmed, and rightly so, about the extent of child abuse in general and child sexual abuse specifically. The taboo against speaking about this abuse is being torn open. But as Florence Rush states in her article "Child Pornography," "We do not have a history of taboos against the sexual use of children."[10] It is important to understand that the phenomenon of violence against women and children and the condoning of this violence is not simply a contemporary perversion but part of an ancient and pervasive worldwide tradition.

10. Florence Rush, "Child Pornography," in *Take Back the Night: Women on Pornography,* ed. Laura Lederer (New York: William Morrow, 1980), p. 71.

In biblical times, sex was sanctioned between men and young girls.[11] Under talmudic law, the sexual use of girls over the age of three was permissible, provided the girl's father consented and appropriate moneys were transferred. Sexual intercourse was an acceptable means of establishing betrothal, and the use of both women and girls was regulated by a detailed set of laws reflecting the property status of females. Women and girls were owned, rented, bought, and sold as sexual commodities. As long as these transactions were conducted with proper payment to the males, rabbis and lawmakers approved.

The sexual use of girls under the age of three was not regulated legally, as these children were considered too young to be legal virgins, and were therefore without monetary value. Sex with girls under the age of three was not subject to any restrictions. As in hunting, it was open season. Boys under the age of nine were also fair game. Though sex between adult men was severely punished, men could—and did—use young boys at will.

The advent of Christianity did not change things substantially. Canon law held that sexual intercourse established possession, and popes through the centuries upheld rape as an indissoluble means of contracting a marriage. However, Christian law raised the age for legally valid sex from three to seven, making sexual intercourse with girls over seven binding and sexual intercourse

---

11. Florence Rush, *The Best Kept Secret*, pp. 16–47. Rush documents abuse through biblical, talmudic, and Christian eras. Her research is detailed and stunning, providing historical validation for these terrible realities. I am indebted to her for the following information and invite those of you who want to know more to read *The Best Kept Secret* and to investigate Rush's sources. For her chapter on the Bible and the Talmud, she cites, among others, *The Babylonian Talmud*, Seder Nezikin, ed.; *The Book of Women*, Moses Maimonides; *The Mishna*, Eugene J. Lipman, ed.; *Marital Relations, Birth Control, and Abortion in Jewish Law*, David M. Feldman; *Sex Laws and Customs in Judaism*, Louis M. Epstein; and the Old Testament itself. For the Christians, she cites, among others, *History of Sacerdotal Celibacy in the Christian Church*, Henry Charles Lea; *Medieval Panorama*, G.G. Coulton; *The Matrimonial Impediment of Nonage*, John C. O'Dea; *Marriage Legislation in the New Code of Canon Law*, Rev. H. A. Ayrinhac; *Medieval Civilization in Western Europe*, V.H.H. Green; and *Laws of Marriage*, John Fulton.

with girls under seven of no consequence to the authorities. In the thirteenth century, the concept of statutory rape was introduced. Its enforcement was not impressive, however, as the clergy itself infamously exploited girls sexually—in the confessional and in the convent schools.

In India, for centuries, marriages have been arranged between men, often old men, and young girls. By the age of ten or twelve, sometimes much younger, the girl-child is forced to submit to intercourse. She is subjected to the physical pain and sometimes permanent injury that repeated intercourse wreaks on a child. The child does not wish for her husband's death, however, since she may be killed when he dies. For centuries, the widow-child was forced to burn herself upon her husband's funeral pyre. This practice, *suttee,* though legally banned for over a century and no longer common, is still in existence.[12]

For a thousand years, girl children in China were compelled to undergo the excruciating pain of foot binding. This torturous process reduced the feet to three- or four-inch stumps—feet the size of a baby's—which became infected and putrefied, sometimes to the extent that toes dropped off. Tiny feet were crucial to marriage, and marriage was crucial to economic survival. Men found the tiny, childlike, mutilated feet sexually attractive. This process began at age five or six or seven.[13]

12. This information is from Mary Daly, *Gyn/Ecology* (Boston: Beacon Press, 1978), pp. 113–33.

13. This information is from Mary Daly, *Gyn/Ecology,* pp. 134–52, and Andrea Dworkin, *Woman Hating* (New York: E.P. Dutton, 1974), pp. 95–117. (In *Woman Hating,* Andrea Dworkin has a small section on incest in which she advocates the destruction of the incest taboo as being "essential to the development of cooperative human community based on the free-flow of natural androgynous eroticism." Because I know her as a pioneer in the exposure of violence toward women and children, I wrote to her asking whether she would send me a clarifying statement or disclaimer to include in this reference. She replied, "I hope some day I will be able to figure out how what we call 'the incest taboo' functions to, in fact, sanction especially father-daughter rape.... The problem is the nature of sexuality in this male-supremacist system, so that all the love, sensuality, and curiosity of children ends up being cynically used against them, in sex as in so many other areas. So I do not advocate incest; and I do speak out against it, naming it the sexual abuse of children. It has become one of my priority concerns.")

In many African countries today and on other continents in the past, girl children have been subjected to the atrocities of genital mutilation, excision, and infibulation. These processes include cutting away the clitoris, inner labia, and parts of the outer labia, then closing the vulva again, leaving an opening for urine. No anesthetic, no antiseptic—the knife may be broken glass, the closing may be thorns, or sometimes the vulva is scraped and the child's legs tied together for weeks until the wound adheres. Often she becomes infected; sometimes she dies. When she marries, she is cut again for intercourse; for childbirth again. The cutting and resewing continue. This process begins as early as several weeks after birth or as late as adolescence. Organizations such as UNICEF and the United Nations Children's Commission have been unwilling to speak out against such tortures because, they say, they do not wish to interfere with native customs.[14]

In every war, along with the glorified killing of men by men, the women and children are also raped, tortured, and killed. This is cross-cultural: Cossacks raped Jewish children, Pakistanis raped Bengali children, Americans raped Vietnamese children, Germans raped French children.[15]

In Europe, between the late 1400s and late 1800s, an estimated nine million people were murdered as witches, most of them women and girls. With the full support of the Christian church, they were gang-raped, tortured with horrendous instruments, forced to confess to sexual crimes, maimed, and burned alive. Commonly, women and girls as young as five were accused of copulation with the devil. Sometimes the girls were so abused they believed it *was* the devil who tormented them. In a manner of speaking, it was.[16]

14. Mary Daly, *Gyn/Ecology*, pp. 153–77.
15. This information is from Susan Brownmiller, *Against Our Will*, pp. 23–130.
16. This information is from Barbara Ehrenreich and Deirdre English, *Witches, Midwives, and Nurses: A History of Women Healers* (Old Westbury, N.Y.: The Feminist Press, 1973); Mary Daly, *Gyn/Ecology*, pp. 178–222; Andrea Dworkin, *Woman Hating*, pp. 118–50; Florence Rush, *The Best Kept Secret*, pp. 37–43.

In America today, juvenile prisons incarcerate children who have committed no crime but whose parents want them off their hands. Seventy percent of these are girls. Often they will be raped by sheriff, coroner, or attendants.[17]

The sexual abuse of girls spans centuries and continents. It is perpetrated by men, either directly, as in rape, or through women as pawns. In China, for example, foot binding was administered by women. However, it was not they who originated the idea. Men created the horror of foot binding; men found it erotic that women should be maimed, suffering, and homebound. Women complied because a bound foot was the only way to insure a daughter's marriage and thus economic and literal survival. The same is true of genital mutilation. The same is true when a mother will not let herself see that her daughter is being molested by her husband. Sometimes she is afraid of the loss of economic support, sometimes she is afraid of further physical violence to herself or her children. Sometimes she is afraid of something much more vague, but just as real—confronting the momentum of an old and deeply embodied attitude that allows men the privilege of ownership and desecration.

We Are in Danger

In this volume, we say no to that desecration. We look clearly at what sexual abuse and rape have meant in these women's lives. We do not avert our eyes to avoid the pain. Statistics, for all the horror they imply, can be so vast that we shield ourselves from the individual lives they represent. We wanted to make the statistics real, to present the pain of the individual. At times the enormity overwhelmed us. It is not easy to open oneself to the knowledge that millions of children are raped. Our defenses rush

17. Vera Goodman, "Juvenile Detention for Girls a Horror," *New Directions for Women* 8, no. 3 (Summer 1979), pp. 7-8.

to protect us from experiencing that pain. But we cannot close ourselves off and hope for the best. We are in danger. Our daughters are in danger. Even our sons are in danger. Behind each statistic, there is a child. She may be you. She may be your daughter. She may be your sister. She may be your friend. You cannot protect her until we can protect all children.

Advertisements, Media, Pornography

Advertisements, the media, and pornography encourage acceptance of the sexual use of children. By blurring the distinction between woman and girl-child, these omnipresent images sometimes leave the message that children, as well as women, can be—and should be—sexually consumed. Women are photographed in seductive poses dressed in ankle socks, holding lollipops and teddy bears. Adolescent and preadolescent girls are photographed soft-focus in and out of lacy, ribboned lingerie.

David Hamilton is one of the best-known photographers of this kind. The preface to his book, *David Hamilton's Private Collection*, introduces his photographs of young girls in various stages of undress as "moments when innocence and eroticism mingle." In one photograph a young girl lies on her stomach, her illuminated buttocks exposed. The caption reads: "To what caresses, pleasures, and mischiefs do you thus offer your perfect and obedient body?" [18]

In one month, December 1981, I bought four widely distributed men's magazines: *Playboy, Oui, Gallery,* and *Hustler.* Each had at least one reference to sex with children, either explicit or an innuendo.

Gallery announced a nude photography contest with a photo of a woman dressed only in socks and roller skates, her hair in pigtails, holding a child's school composition book in mittened

18. *David Hamilton's Private Collection* (New York: Morrow Quill, 1980).

hands. In *Oui,* a letter to the editor asked, "Would it be possible to have your models wear white ankle socks and saddle shoes?" In the same issue, as part of a "Celebrity Sex Lives" quiz, readers were invited to guess who said "I have never been able to understand how a father could tenderly love his charming daughter without having slept with her at least once." *Playboy* printed a cartoon in which a little girl on Santa's knee asks for ben-wa balls, body lotion, and a talking vibrator and then says, "Mm, your knee feels nice! I just adore older men." *Hustler* advertised "Little Magazines and Movies," offering men the chance to look at children being sexually exploited by adults. Other times *Hustler* cartoons have featured "Chester the Molester," joking about child molestation.

In movies, young girls are portrayed as sexual commodities. Jodie Foster in *Taxi Driver* and Brooke Shields in *Pretty Baby* both play the parts of happy twelve-year-old prostitutes.[19]

The same day I bought the magazines, the *Oakland Tribune* reported that Brooke Shields was in court seeking to block future commercial use of nude photographs made of her when she was ten years old.[20] Under that article was another about a seventeen-year-old runaway who had been sexually abused by adult male friends of his family at age seven. By age fifteen he was a drug-dependent male prostitute. The newspapers have been reporting similar tragedies often over the last few years. The *Minneapolis Star* reported that children are recruited for prostitution in large numbers, that poor tenants in Minneapolis accept money from pimps who use their apartments as "catches" where children are

19. Florence Rush discusses these movies in "Child Pornography," in *Take Back the Night: Women on Pornography,* ed. Laura Lederer (New York: William Morrow, 1980), pp. 74–75.

20. The *Oakland Tribune,* November 6, 1981, p. A-3. (In a statement representative of the conflicting messages this society gives girls and women, the judge said both that Brooke Shields's mother shouldn't have allowed the pictures to be taken and that there was nothing wrong with the pictures. He ruled against blocking future commercial use.)

broken in before being shipped to New York or Chicago.[21]

The *Los Angeles Times* estimated that "one and a half million children under sixteen are used annually in commercial sex (prostitution or pornography)."[22] In 1977, *Time* magazine reported that the child pornography industry had become a billion-dollar-a-year business.[23] By now the actual figures can only be worse. In San Francisco, at a child's eye level, newspaper vending machines feature tabloids of prostitution and pornography. The cover of the issue I picked up portrayed a young woman's body with a childlike face and long hair in pigtails. The face could have been that of a twelve-year-old. Inside, along with much advertisement for adult sex, there were also ads for movies and magazines that sexually exploit children, such as *Nasty Playmate, Lollipop Pet,* and *Wanna See My P.P.* The price: "$2.00 per tiny tot."

The record industry uses sex and violence against children for profit. The British cover of *Virgin Killers* by the group Scorpion shows a little girl with broken glass projecting from her vagina.[24] Though that album cover is now banned in the United States, the group continues to distribute other albums here with covers consistently degrading to women.

On the cover of Rachel Sweet's album *Protect the Innocent,* a woman dressed in a black leather jacket and black gloves wraps her hands around the mouth and nose of a child, leaving only the child's eyes exposed.

The portrayal of women and girls on record albums ranges from explicitly violent to insipidly degrading. One cover shows woman-girl as cake: the white iced cake, complete with eyes,

21. The *Minneapolis Star,* March 19, 1981, p. 8-A.
22. Statistics from "Children—A Big Profit Item from the Smut Producers," John Hurst, *Los Angeles Times,* May 26, 1977, in Florence Rush, "Child Pornography," p. 77.
23. *Time,* April 1977.
24. Copies of this album were destroyed by members of the Preying Mantis Women's Brigade of Santa Cruz, California, a group dedicated to ending violence against women and children.

mouth, arms, and legs, swinging on a garden swing, one piece sliced from between her legs, exposing the chocolate inside. A man watches from the corner behind her.

Hartman's Heart Breakers, a 1930s reprint of hillbilly songs sung by Betty Lou, shows a drawing of an old man fiddler leering at a woman-girl with huge breasts, a bow in her hair, and panties showing under a short, little-girl skirt. She leans into him with the caption, "Give it to me, Daddy." On the back it says, "Prepare your ears for an apparent 11-year-old elucidating the pleasure of mattresses, springs, How to Diddle and Shake That Thing. Betty Lou's voice lies somewhere between those of Shirley Temple, Baby Rose Marie, and a Tennessee Williams wanton." Quoting from the songs, the blurb ends with, "Daddy, O Daddy, don't be so mean! Reach up on the shelf and get the Vaseline."

Even television advertisements convey the message that little girls are sexually available. One ad for a major mattress company showed a little girl curled up on the mattress. The caption, in large black letters, read: "Try something new." And in an ad for a department store, a little girl tries on frilly dresses for her daddy, posing coyly, with the narration, "For the man in her life."

Jokes about child sexual abuse abound. A couple of years ago, a major cosmetics company introduced a new shade of nail polish called "Statutory Grape." Only after widespread feminist protest did they drop the name.

Linda Lee Curns, author of "Sittin Pidgins," a story about a child who outwits a molester, wrote that she was repeatedly told, "A Tennessee virgin is a girl who can outrun her brothers."[25] One man who had molested his stepdaughter and is now involved with Parents United told us he'd heard many times growing up, "Old enough to bleed, old enough to slaughter." He also told another so-called joke: "A guy comes home and says, 'Pa, I'm in

---

25. Linda Lee Curns's story is one of the many excellent submissions we were not able to include due to space limitations.

love. I found a virgin and I want to marry her.' The old man says, 'A virgin? How old is she?' 'She's twelve.' 'Good grief! Doesn't she have any brothers?' 'Yes, she's got six brothers.' 'Well, I'm sorry but you can't marry her.' 'Why not?' 'If she's not good enough for her own kin, she's not good enough for us.'"

Several years ago I was at a Halloween party. One man walked in dressed in a raincoat. Upon opening the coat, he revealed a long salami sticking out of his fly. Almost everyone there thought it was funny—or pretended to. They were unaware that joking about men exposing their genitals is a way of condoning that behavior and ignoring the real damage done to children.

Though child molestation is ostensibly condemned, it is in actuality sanctioned by our institutions, by movies, magazines, advertising, even art and literature.[26] All of these confuse adult women with children; vulnerability with sexual invitation; masculinity with aggression; yes with no; women with their genitals; and both women and children with property, owned by men.

Men are taught to equate power and violence with a sense of well-being. Many seek this sense of well-being so desperately, so recklessly, that they are willing to look for it even in the bodies of children. Their concern for the child is too weak to check them, their desire for domination too strong.

Violence to Life

In a world that is polluted, possibly beyond recovery, and in which the health of future generations is mortgaged for cars and electrical appliances, it is perfectly consistent that so many men foul the lives of children. It reflects a deep selfishness, an insistence that their desires be met, at whatever cost to others, even to their own children.

The sexual abuse of children is part of a culture in which violence to life is condoned. Our forests, our rivers, our oceans, our

26. For more examples, see Florence Rush, *The Best Kept Secret.*

air, our earth, this entire biosphere, all are invaded with poison—raped, just as our children are raped. It is very possible that in fifty years or less, life as we know it will not exist on earth. Nuclear war could kill us all. Even without an explosion, the radiation emitted in the various phases of mining, milling, and constructing nuclear power plants and weapons is already so abundant that the continuation of our species is in grave danger.[27] It is not odd that men whose desire for profit has superseded their own instinct for survival should so abuse their young. To stunt a child's trust in people, in love, in her world, to instill a fear that may take a lifetime to overcome, may never be overcome, to force one's body into the body of a child, of a baby, to desecrate children so is consistent for people who desecrate all life and the possibility of future life.[28]

He Violates the Child

What is happening in the minds of men who perpetrate this destruction? What is happening in the minds of men who sexually

27. For information on the threat to all life on earth from nuclear power and nuclear war, see Helen Caldicott, *Nuclear Madness* (New York: Bantam, 1981); Anna Gyorgy and Friends, *No Nukes: Everyone's Guide to Nuclear Power* (Boston: South End Press, 1979); and John W. Gofman, *Irrevy: An Irreverent Illustrated View of Nuclear Power* (Committee for Nuclear Responsibility, Main P.O. Box 11207, San Francisco, California 94101, 1979).

28. Leading scientists and physicians from the most prestigious universities, Nobel laureates, and those who have held key positions in the nuclear industry judge that we live in immediate danger of annihilating all life on earth. The clock of the *Bulletin of the Atomic Scientists,* "Symbol of the threat of nuclear doomsday," stands at four minutes to midnight. Four minutes until the end of the world.

The Pentagon talks of "acceptable" numbers of deaths. The vice president of the United States, George Bush, says on television that nuclear war is not unthinkable; that we must think about it; that even if only 10,000 Americans survived, it would still be a victory. This is clearly a man split from his feeling, a man split from his body. And he is not alone. (Since this statement, made in the spring of 1981, others in key positions in the U.S. government have made similar insane and terrifying public statements.) He is not an aberration. Just as a child rapist is not alone. He acts like a monster. But he is not a monster. Somewhere, beneath the monster, is a human person. The question is, Can and will enough of these humans find their integrated human natures, own their nature, love nature, before they destroy themselves and the rest of life?

abuse children? One woman who, as a girl, was repeatedly raped by her father recalled asking him, "Why are you doing this to me?" He answered, "I wish I knew." Some men are not so honest about their ignorance. They say—and often have convinced themselves—that they are "teaching" the child, or they "need" the child's body, or it's their "right." But their pathetic stature (as in Jude Brister's portrayal of her father at the end of "The Window's Netting"), their authoritarianism (as in "These Are the Things I Remember" by Maggie Hoyal), and their dependency and infantilism (as in "California Daughter" by Jean Monroe), show the extent to which men are out of control—out of touch with their feelings, out of touch with whatever their authentic needs might be. This irony: that from their being out of touch with themselves, they touch the child. These men look outward to the child for what they lack so desperately in themselves.

The man violates the child. He violates the innocence, the clarity, the authenticity of the child. He violates the body still in its original knowledge of itself, before it experiences responding to another. He violates the simplicity of the body, the child's body, her tenderness, her vulnerability, her trust. And more, he violates the child in himself—his own tenderness, his body, his feelings for himself, his original idea of himself, before he was told he was a monster, before he was told he was violent, must act violent, before he was told men rape women, overpower women, before he was told he was a man. He violates himself, his home, his world.

He does not know why. He does not know his own mind or his own body. He is a stranger to himself. And because he does not know himself, does not feel himself, he has in effect given himself up. There is no self to withstand the onslaught of messages he receives from his culture, encouraging him to abuse children.

I recently went to a meeting of Parents United. I asked the group of men who had molested children, their own daughters and step-daughters, "What made it okay? Do you know where you got the message that it was okay for you to molest a child?" One man agreed to talk with me.

"I was molested as a child myself," he said. "My wife was molested as a child also." Many men who were molested as children go on to molest their own children. Women rarely molest children. Even though many more girls than boys are molested, very few women inflict sexual abuse on their children. However, when women are taught through rape and molestation that they have no rights to their bodies, and when, in growing up, they do not gain the strength to reclaim these rights, they sometimes allow men into their lives who do not respect women or children and, not knowing how to protect themselves, these women do not know how to protect their daughters either.

The man went on. "I remember the feeling I had of disgust . . . I felt that if I was a really good person, this would not have happened. And with my uncle I really felt weakness and helplessness." He was beaten. "I never had any rights. I didn't even have the rights to my feelings." He did not know a reason for the beatings. "Now I've figured out that I was getting beaten for expressing individuality . . . but then all I was aware of was sometimes I got a beating for being too noisy and other times for being too quiet." As a child he undressed with another child. The mother of the child called him "a little monster." "And this woman . . . it was obvious that my family was holding me down because I had done something wrong, because they were right and I was wrong. And this woman kind of explained what was wrong with me. That really stuck in my mind and I think that's part of what made it okay. *I'm a monster.*"

He was told rape was okay, a tradition. "My stepfather's stepfather got busted for having a thirteen-year-old girl in the trailer with him. He was a traveling minister and it was one of those things that people were smiling about—because he was a minister. . . . We caught him. There was an undercurrent in the back, an implication that everybody does it." He was told "sex was nasty and everyone did it and no part of it was good." He learned molestation was adventurous. "There was this girl from San Francisco whose father was a member of the Beat Generation and they had spent the summer down in Brazil and Kerouac went with them. She had shared with me that Kerouac had oral sex with her when she was eight." This impressed him. He admired this man. "He was one of the people who had made it without compromising his talent and his beliefs."

He felt weak. He felt out of control of his life. As a child he was sent to live with a cousin, a grandfather, an aunt and uncle. His father was gone. His mother was an alcoholic. He felt worthless. "I had to express my power over people," he said, "I *felt* so powerless." He fought his feelings of inadequacy by forcing his stepdaughter to submit to sex. "See, I'm not really weak. I can make *you* do something."

This man's feelings were denied in childhood. He did not know his feelings. He was afraid to feel. "It was when I got into this program that I began to understand that I had feelings and that I was responsible for them. It was such a revelation." He took part in an exercise. The leader instructed the group to express feelings without using words. "You're angry," she said. "You're mad at everybody and everything including yourself." Then, "You're so smug." Then, "You're depressed." Last, "You're in love." He acted out these feelings. He grimaced, he sighed. "I was aware," he said, "of a change in my own feelings. Sure, I was following her voice. But *I* was the one who did it!"

He began to feel again. He could bear feelings, even feelings of powerlessness. "At times I've felt real powerless . . . and the way I've handled that is that it's probably a temporary thing . . . when I get off probation, I'll probably start getting some of that power back. But right now everyone's got power over me. . . . It's just a fact." He could bear feelings of pain, loss, fear. "Scary. Really scary. At times some of the changes that I've made are so sweeping that I've felt like I was becoming an entirely different person. And I felt like I was dying because the person I had been was no longer." And he began to create his own power. He was no longer afraid of being known. "Right now there's nothing in my life that I feel I have to keep hidden."

He has regained a sense of his own self. "I think I'm developing a lot of inner strength. An understanding of things makes me feel more accepting, more separate, more unique. And yet more like everybody else because even though I'm feeling more unique, my understanding is that everybody's unique. Intellectually, it seems confusing. Emotionally, I can really see it." He joins humanity. He is no longer a monster. He is a human being.[29]

This man has been willing to admit his guilt, to ask forgiveness, to work to understand himself. He has made a commitment to respect his daughter. He speaks in schools, telling young people that they have the right to protect themselves against sexual abuse, encouraging them to ask for help if they need it. He tells them he molested his daughter; that he was wrong, that no one, not even a parent, has the right to use a child sexually.[30]

Although this man is not alone, it is still extremely rare for men who have molested children to recognize and assume full responsibility for the pain and suffering they have inflicted. Nothing— not apologies, not tears, not anguish or attempts to make up for what has been done—nothing can undo the betrayal that a violated child has suffered. But if the molester sincerely admits his guilt

29. I am indebted to Susan Griffin here for the influence of her work. Her book *Pornography and Silence: Culture's Revenge Against Nature* (New York: Harper & Row, 1981) made it possible for me to understand more of the process of how a person can be so alienated from life that he can violate a child.

30. I want to thank the members of the Santa Cruz Parents United group for allowing me to attend their meeting. I want especially to thank this man who told us his story for his time and effort. I think the work of Parents United is valuable. However, when the editors of *I Never Told Anyone* held a local reading from the book (announcing it at a Parents United meeting), although a number of women came, the only male to attend from Parents United was a boy who had been molested. Not one man from this group came to hear what women had to say.

and asks forgiveness, if he commits himself to change and responsibility, sometimes this can contribute to the healing journey the child must undertake to regain her whole, vital self.

The Gift of Anger

Only once as a child was I approached sexually by a man. The incident was minor, but I include it here because my mother's reaction was so strong and affirming of my personhood, my dignity, that I feel it is an example worth sharing.

I was eleven. We had just moved from our apartment over my parents' liquor store to a house with a small yard. Ted, one of the men who worked in the store, had finished mowing our grass and came into the house for a cold soda. My grandmother was in the kitchen, making dinner; my parents were at work; I was teaching myself to type in what we called the "recreation room," just off the kitchen. My older brother had made me a chart of the keyboard, showing which fingers to use on which keys, and I was practicing on an old black metal machine, typing from the *Golden Book Encyclopedia*. Ted walked into the room and said, "Typing, huh?"

We had lived over the store for ten years. The men who worked there were my friends. They drove me to playmates' houses in the delivery truck. One let me sit on his lap and help steer. One went fast over the railroad tracks to make my stomach flip-flop. I spent Saturday nights in the store eating sno-cones and reading comic books while my parents answered the phone, slipped pints and fifths into brown paper bags, rang up sales on the register. Sometimes I helped fill in the refrigerator with cans of beer and soda, and I loved to dust the tiny bottles of maraschino cherries.

Ted was new, but I had no experience that would cause me to be wary. "I'm practicing," I said. "Learning to do it without looking at the keys."

"Hey, that's pretty good," he said. "Look out the window. See how the grass is all filling in. I did a pretty nice job, huh?"

I stood up and looked. "That's great," I said. We had never had grass before, or a regular house with a doorbell that people rang and you went to the door to answer it. Everyone had always entered through the store. So I was delighted at all the accouterments of a real house.

"How about giving me a kiss for doing such a good job?" He smiled at me.

I was surprised by his request, but I didn't want to offend him. I'd kissed uncles and family friends plenty of times. It was a form of politeness. So I leaned toward him to give a peck on the cheek.

He wrapped his arms around me, pulled me to him, and shoved his tongue into my mouth. I stood there stunned for a moment, and when he loosened his hold, I ran out of the room, upstairs to the bathroom, and locked myself in. I sat on the closed toilet seat, holding on to the blue towel hanging from the rack, deciding not to come out until I was sure he was gone and my mother had returned, deciding not to tell my mother. I was afraid she'd blame me.

Eventually he left and my mother came home, calling out, "Hello, it's robbers," her well-worn joke. Hearing her voice, my resolve not to tell melted and I called weakly, "Mom, I'm upstairs. Could you come up a minute?"

I was crying before I even started talking and she sat me down on my bed, sitting next to me with her coat still on, her arms around me, saying, "What is it, Ellen? What happened?"

I told her, haltingly.

"The bastard," she hissed, and I felt something break free in me. "The bastard, the son of a bitch," she repeated. "I'm sorry you didn't bite his tongue off, poke his eyes out. You should have hollered for Grandmom. The two of you could have beat him up." She held me and her anger washed me clean. I was innocent. There was no longer a doubt. I was innocent.

The next day when she came home from work, she told me what had happened there. When Ted walked into the store, she said to him, "You have guts to come back here."

"What do you mean?" he asked.

"I mean if you ever touch Ellen again, I'll tell your wife. If you see her on the street, cross and walk on the other side."

"I didn't do anything," he protested. He needed the job. "I only kissed her."

He had a five-year-old daughter. My mother asked, "How would you like it if Mr. Bass kissed your daughter that way?"

The man blanched. My mother fired him. I never saw him again.

My mother gave me the gift of anger, the strength and healing power of fury and direct action. My mother believed me, she vindicated me, she protected me. I learned I could protect myself. I was not prey. I felt safe. Relatively.

I was still afraid of walking home alone at night, shadows, dark bushes, even the dark upstairs when I went to my room alone. But these fears did not stem from my personal experience; rather, our culture, the real dangers of our world, seep into our minds at an early age. We learn fear even before we know how much there truly is to fear. We learn shame, degradation, humiliation, and we learn these things have something to do with sex, with men and women, with our bodies, our own selves.

Twisted Images

Working on this anthology has brought me into conscious struggle with the twisted, deep-rooted images of myself as a sexual female that I have absorbed from my environment through my life. Distorted, disturbing images I have suppressed have barged into my consciousness, upsetting me, forcing me to confront how I have been warped.

As I read and reread the stories of women who had been raped and abused, there were times when I could not bear to be touched. Too many stories of too many fingers, tongues, penises of adult men slipping into little girls' vaginas made it impossible for me to open my body to a man. I lost interest in sex. I did not recognize why. I was distressed. I wanted to share intimacy, but when I began to make love, I'd feel the halted breath of little girls trying not to breathe, stiffening, hoping the large invasive hand would disappear, wanting to disappear themselves. Or I'd fantasize other lovers, ones I knew before I knew about child molestation, ones who lived far away, so I need not confront real hands on my real body. Or I would be distracted by an image of myself as a stripper, gyrating in a dark theater in front of ogling men. This picture disgusted me. I didn't understand it. I hated that it was a part of my mind. Then I remembered:

When I was a small child, my mother took me to the doctor. I don't remember what for. In the examining room, I took off my clothes. I don't know whether I misunderstood the directions about what clothes to remove, whether I seemed cheerful about disrobing, or whether the doctor (who liked to pat the bottoms of girls and women alike) said something that elicited this response from my mother, but she laughed and joked, "She's going to be a striptease artist when she grows up."

I was horribly embarrassed. Although I was no older than six or seven, I already knew that a striptease artist was a woman who took off her clothes for the sexual pleasure of men. And although I had never seen a stripper, and the only pictures I might have looked at were the kind that *Life* magazine could have printed of Las Vegas performers in lavish feathers and sequins, I was enough a child of our culture to feel degradation and shame.

A good girl, I began to guard carefully against the possibility that anyone might think I *wanted* to be seen naked. After a day at the beach when my mother wanted to take off my wet bathing suit in the back of the car, I refused. When she insisted, I said I wouldn't change unless she did. I was not going to risk indiscre-

tion again. I rode home wet and gritty. Now, twenty-five years
later, the stripper reappears, a twisted ghost of a twisted culture.

The more I have examined my own past and listened to the
stories of my sisters, the more I have remembered: pornographic
magazines my father hid in our garage; playing cards with pictures of women in provocative poses. And way back, the calendar
in the candy store. I was allowed to walk there myself, carefully
crossing two streets, waiting on the high leather stool while the
old man mixed me a chocolate malted to take home. There were
brown chocolate and white chocolate bunnies at Easter, big coco-
nut-cream-filled eggs with sugar ribbons and flowers on top. He
made the candy himself. The smell was heavenly. Above the mix-
er where my milkshake was whirring hung a calendar. The picture: a woman holding groceries in both arms, her back to me, but
she looked over her shoulder right at me, her mouth a surprised
red O, her underpants having slipped down to her ankles, wind
blowing up her skirt, her rosy buttocks exposed. The style of the
painting was Norman Rockwell: the youth and health of the
woman, her winsome dismay at her plight, all construed to present a feeling of fun, of pleasure. But even in this "innocent"
cheesecake are the elements of degradation. The woman is helpless, her arms are full. She cannot pull up her pants, push down
her skirt, walk or run. The viewer, presumably, is chuckling, enjoying his view of her, enjoying her "appealing" dismay as well as
her nakedness.

Who buys candy, ice-cream sodas, and chocolate bunnies? How
many little girls and boys sat looking at that calendar? The old
man behind the counter never touched my body and he may not
have touched the bodies of the other children either. But the
picture embeds. Notice, next time you are shopping, the covers of
magazines at children's eye level.

As a small child—I couldn't have been more than eight; perhaps as young as five or six—I played with two sisters, one three
years older than I, one a year younger. We played together almost

every day, all kinds of games and make-believe, among them a play we'd act out, which we called "King and Slave Girl." The oldest sister was the king. I was the slave girl. The youngest was the castle guard. She would bring me to the king, whose lap I would sit on while she fondled my flat breasts beneath my T-shirt. I was not forced by these sisters into this game, rather, we were all forced into it by what we had absorbed from our world. We lived out the sadistic pornography that had already infiltrated our consciousness.

I was not sexually abused. Yet I was sexually abused. We were all sexually abused. The images and attitudes, the reality we breathe in like air, it reaches us all. It shapes and distorts us, prunes some of our most tender, trusting, lovely and loving branches. We learn that this is who a woman is. This is what men think of women. This is what we are taught to think about ourselves.

We all, women and men, live our lives in an environment that fouls one of the magnificent, holy aspects of our natural world. Creation, love, fertility, the union of two becoming one, joining in body and in ecstasy—this possibility, which should be our birthright, has been fouled. We are all wounded. We all need healing.

My own healing has been and continues to be a difficult but rewarding journey. When I finally remembered the incident in the doctor's office, the image of the stripper lost its grip. It no longer insinuated its way into my mind. I could let it go. When I admitted to myself the depth of the revulsion I felt for what men have done to children, when I let myself see clearly the blatant and sly ways men have used women and children for their own ends, I released the possibility of seeing that sometimes, at least sometimes, men come to women with integrity.

Recently I have recognized that the image of the stripper is a perverted travesty of a basic and vital impulse—the desire to be seen, to be known, naked, in sexual sharing. The reason that image had power for me was that it expressed, though in a deeply distorted way, this essential and exciting aspect of sexuality—that of showing oneself, revealing oneself, and being accepted. When I realized this, I was overwhelmed with feelings: anger and sadness at the insidiousness of our culture's effect on our lives; relief in finally understanding why such ugliness was a part of me; and exhilaration at reclaiming the erotic strength and vigor of the original desire, that of sharing who I truly am with my lover, both as a gift and as an affirmation of my self.

We Can Teach Our Children

Validating Our Children's Integrity

June 1980
Sara at two

Some time ago I was shopping with my child. I sat her on the check-out counter while I got my money. The cashier reached over and tickled her leg. For one second she sat perfectly still, then her face contorted and she cried. I picked her up and spoke softly: "There, there, you don't need to be afraid, don't cry, he was just wanting to make you laugh, he didn't mean to make you cry." In the safety of my arms, she was comforted. I smiled briefly at the cashier and we left with our packages.

For a long time the incident stayed in the back of my mind, while now and then similar incidents, in other stores, at the houses of friends, occurred. Each time my response was the same: I'd soothe her, tell her it was all right—the person hadn't meant to upset her. Then one day, after I had been working on this book, another cashier greeted my daughter and touched her leg. She began to cry and I picked her up as before, but this time I told her, "You can say *no,* you can say *don't touch me.* You know how to say that." Between short catches of breath, nuzzled into my shoulder, she mumbled "No."

The next time she will say *no* louder. And I will tell the cashier,

"She doesn't want to be touched." Soon she'll say clearly, in her high voice, "I not want be touch." The cashier may laugh at her seriousness, but I will not laugh. Driving home, I will tell her, "That's good. That's good how you told the person in the store not to touch you. I don't like people to touch me that way either."

Yet this will not assure her safety. A rapist could still assault her with force; a man she knows well could approach her with mock tenderness and she could misunderstand, become confused, panic into submission. All this is possible until men learn the difference between love and violation, intimacy and domination, filling one's own needs and limitless selfishness; until their greed for power is replaced by compassion and they learn to nurture the young, each other, women, themselves. Until then, she is not safe. But this is a start. An essential start.

We can teach our children to respect themselves, to trust their feelings, to trust their inner voice. We can teach our children their dignity, their worth, their ability to discriminate. We must learn these things ourselves so we can teach them to our children.

Her Own Power

January 1981
Sara at two and a half

One day, Sara and I were grocery shopping. One of the workers in the store likes to make jokes with her. She likes his jokes, but is also afraid. He is tall, wears brightly colored hats, talks fast and loud. At a distance she enjoys his teasing, but when he touched her, though it was a light pat on the head, she ran crying to me, followed by the surprised man.

I picked her up, soothed her, and told the man she was a little afraid of him.

"Of me?" he laughed, astonished. "I'm just a silly old man!"

Still in my arms, Sara turned to him.

"I'm just a silly old man," he laughed again. "You don't have to be afraid of me."

Then she laughed, too. The rest of the day she talked happily about the "silly old man." "But I don't like him to touch me," she told me.

"You can tell him, then," I taught her. "You can say, 'I don't like you to touch me, but I like you to make jokes with me.'"

Sara laughed and demanded, "Again."

Again I said to the imaginary man, "I don't like you to touch me, but I like you to make jokes with me."

Again she laughed, and we did it again and again. Soon she was instructing the man herself, "I don't want you to touch me, but I like to make a joke with you."

The next time we went to the store, the man was filling in produce as we were putting oranges in our cart. He reached out to her and she said, softly and a bit mumbled, but strongly enough to stop him, "I don't want you to touch me, but I like to make a joke with you."

"You don't want me to touch you when you're making a joke with me?" he asked, not quite understanding all her words.

"She's saying she doesn't want you to touch her, but she likes you to make jokes with her," I translated.

"Oh," he said, stepping back one step, his eyebrows raised, a slight, thoughtful smile on his face. "I can understand that. That's okay." He nodded a couple of times, almost to himself, taking this information in. Then he turned back to his work, humming a jazzy tune.

This week when we entered the store, Sara looked all around. "He's not here," she announced, disappointed.

"No, I don't see him," I agreed. "Maybe he's in the back and will come out."

Sure enough, just as we were gathering up our bags, he did come out. "Hi!" she said to him enthusiastically.

"Hi!" he said. "How you doin', huh?" He grinned at her.

She looked at me. "He didn't touch me," she said, surprised.

"No, of course I didn't touch you." He laughed loudly. "You told me not to, didn't you?"

Sara just smiled, allowing this experience of her own power and the world's response to fill her. The man chuckled, pleased with himself. I beamed, proud, hopeful.[31]

"Well, then, I should thank you for your work"

June 1982
Sara at four

It's Sara's fourth birthday party. We're in our friend's large yard, two doors down from our new house. By the end of the party, Sara has deposited her clothes about in the grass and is enjoying the hot sun. She has always hated clothes. Winters I fight with her to put on shoes, a sweater at least. By summer I give up.

"I'm going home to get my Barbie doll," she announces. She's gotten a package of Barbie accessories—hats, jewelry, shoes—and wants to try it all out.

"Okay," I say, "just put on underpants."

This freedom to travel by herself is new. At the old house, there were no sidewalks. Cars came careening around the country road oblivious to dogs and children. Although her best friend lived only three houses down and across the street, she couldn't walk there herself.

Here she is independent. The first evening she discovered she could find her way, remember the houses, and go alone, she ran back and forth every ten minutes for hours.

"Just put on underpants," I repeat. For the past few days I've been repeating that a lot. I gather crepe paper, plastic forks, Styrofoam cups. The guests have left and the yard holds the pleasant feeling of afterward.

31. I wrote a children's story about this experience, "I Like You to Make Jokes with Me, But I Don't Want You to Touch Me," in *Ms.* magazine, October 1982, and in the *Ms.* book, *Stories for Free Children.*

In a few minutes, Sara returns naked, carrying Barbie.

"Sara, I told you you must wear underpants when you're on the street alone."

"I forgot."

"Well, will you be sure to wear them from now on?"

She is silent.

"Will you remember to wear them from now on?" I ask again.

"I'm thinking," she says.

"Okay," I say, "think about it." I pick popped balloon bits from the grass.

"I'm not sure," Sara says. "I don't think I'll remember."

I sigh. Of course not. I haven't told her why. I don't want to tell her why. I have to tell her why. I don't want to.

"Sara, I think you can't remember because you don't know why I want you to wear underpants."

"I don't know why," she agrees.

"And I think it's hard to remember to do something when you don't know why."

"Yes, it is," she agrees.

"So I think I need to tell you why I want you to wear underpants when you're on the street alone." My logic is accurate. I'm stalling for time.

"Okay," she says.

I take a deep breath and snort it out again. "Well," I begin. "It's like this. Most grown-ups are good people. But there are some grown-ups—this is going to sound crazy, but it's true—there are some big people that if they see a child's vagina or penis, they may want to hurt it. It's a terrible thing and it's crazy and I don't understand it, but it's true, and that's why I want you to wear underpants when you're on the street alone. Because if one of those bad people happens to come along, I don't want him to try to hurt you."

"Why do they want to hurt a child's vagina or penis?" she asks me.

"I really don't know, Sara. I don't understand it myself. But it's true. It's terrible, but it's true. And I don't want anyone to hurt you."

"I don't want anyone to hurt my vagina. Would they hurt my anus, too?"

"I don't want them to hurt any of you. That's why I want you to be safe and wear underpants. You know, Sara, how I've told you that in my work I teach people that they should take good care of children and not hurt them?"

"Yes."

"I tell people that sometimes big people hurt children and that's wrong and that they shouldn't do that. A big person should never hurt a child. In my book I write about that. That's part of my work."

"Well, then," she says, putting her hands on her hips, "I should thank you for your work."

Healing

In this book, survivors of childhood sexual abuse use the power of speech to transform, to fuse secret shame, pain, and anger into a sharp useful tool, common as a kitchen knife, for cutting away lies and deception like rotten fruit, leaving the clean hard pit, that kernel of truth: These insults were inflicted, are inflicted now, every day. The repercussions are deep and lasting. The will to survive is strong, the tenacity and beauty of survival inspiring. We are not alone. We are not to blame. We are innocent, innocent and powerful, worthy of our healing fury, self-love, and love for each other.

My work on this anthology, through all the pain and devastation, has been ultimately healing. As I have lived with these stories in my mind, my heart, my body, as I have dreamed them and awakened from dreams sobbing, as I have worked to share them with others, I have felt how the lives of my sisters are more mine each day. Though I was not personally raped, I am a woman. I am the mother of a daughter. I share in the pain, in the anger, in the healing, and in the creation of a world where children are encouraged and empowered to control their own bodies, to protest, and to ask for help, knowing they will get it. Ultimately, I am sharing in the restoration of a consciousness where the rape of children—as well as the rape of women, of forests, of oceans, of the earth—is a history, to be remembered only to assure it will not begin again.

"I had thought it was over"

SURVIVORS OF SEXUAL ABUSE
BY FATHERS

JUDE BRISTER

"Dear Diary,
Nov. 13, 1969
He said he thought that I liked it. Oh, God, that made me mad!"

Jude Brister was born in 1957 in Oakland, California. When she was three years old, her parents were divorced. Both her father, Lee, and her mother remarried, and Jude and her two brothers visited Lee often in his home. When she was four, he began to molest her, and continued to do so until she was twelve. Five months after the abuse described in the "The Window's Netting," her father, a respected high-school science teacher, collapsed with a heart attack and died at the age of forty-six.

Jude was nineteen when she wrote "The Window's Netting." Later she printed it as a booklet and distributed it in local bookstores. This process enabled her to talk extensively with her brothers and mother about the incest. "I then went to see my stepsister, Sarah, who had lived with my father when we were both between the ages of ten and twelve," she explains. "We met in San Francisco in a stark coffeehouse. I handed her the booklet and said, 'There's something I want to tell you about, but it's hard. . . . ' She read a few lines, then put it down. 'I don't need to read it,' she said. 'The same thing was happening to me.' Later Sarah talked to her sister and we found out that all three of us were being molested by my father in the same period of time, and none of us had known about the others."

Another time of unfolding came around the death of Lee's mother, Neva. "Neva had moved in with her daughter, Edna (Lee's sister and my aunt), for the last years of her life. I had little contact with Neva, not wanting to tell her what her son had done, but finding it hard to communicate with her if I didn't tell. When Grandma Neva died, I wrote Edna to explain why I hadn't kept in touch. Edna called and shared that Neva's father had raped a twelve-year-old deaf girl and that Edna herself had been molested by Neva's brother. This unveiled a long line of sexual abuse in the family—great-grandfather, great-uncle, aunt, stepsisters, myself. And who else was involved? How far back?"

Jude worked as an editor on this anthology. "I want people to start talking about child sexual abuse," she states. "The first place to stop it is in your own family."

The Window's Netting

Carrie is eleven years old traveling with her brother, Keith, and father, Lee, into the mountains of Bear Valley to build a cabin. They drive silent through gold hills. Small, thin, with straight bangs, straight brown hair, the bare beginnings of breasts, Carrie sits in the back seat watching her father drive. She sees his strong hands on the wheel, the black hairs curled around his arm. His soft features that can be so gentle are intent on the road. Leaning forward he is sucking on hard candies, greased black hair combed to the side falling into his face.

Carrie is glad to be with him. Lee chose to have just Keith and her come along on this trip, after a long while of having to share him with his new wife and stepchildren. *He must love us, love me, love us, love me,* the words singsong in her head as the pines begin to sprout on the hills around them. Something troubles her though. She remembers a long time ago, before Lee was remarried . . . but it's been so long, she thinks, been too long for it to happen again.

Lee senses Carrie watching him. "What've you been up to lately?" he asks, glancing back at her in the mirror.

"Oh, not much really." She is jumped out of her thoughts. Smiling carefully, trying not to let her braces glint, she leans forward between the two seats Lee and Keith are sitting in. Keith ignores her, continuing to stare out at cars passing the other way, counting the number of black ones. "I've been playing with my friends and reading a lot. I read um a book, no, two books on the Donner Party."

"Hmmm," says Lee, his eyes back on the road.

"It was funny," Carrie goes on, "they both had the same line in them about . . . no, it's not really funny but both books have chapters that end with . . ." She sees that he isn't listening and sinks back into her seat.

He speeds up to pass a car and Carrie closes her eyes until they are safely in their own lane.

They arrive at the land early in the evening and see the first story of the cabin is built. The stars spangle, they eat a can of beans heated on a Coleman stove, and slowly, as the dark, the black noises thicken around them, they share a Hershey bar. In silence Carrie lets the chocolate melt through on her tongue. Keith, tall like her father, fourteen and withdrawn these days, acne spotting his face, says he wants to sleep alone in a tent beside the cabin. She and Lee are going to sleep in the big tent that is on top of the finished first floor. Tired from a long day of traveling, the sun long down, they head to bed.

The tent is dark and Carrie sits on her sleeping bag, dark green with a silver silky lining. She sits on it putting in the rubber bands for her braces. Sensing Lee is waiting for her to finish putting on her headgear, she takes a long time. They are new braces, they hurt. She has to place a small rubber band, a tight rubber band, from a hook on the top of one tooth to a hook on a bottom tooth. She sees her father out of the corner of her eye, naked, sitting on his sleeping bag, watching; it bothers her. It is dark in the tent. She smells the canvas walls, the plastic floor, and looks straight ahead, concentrating on the rubber bands, saying *Go away, go away* to her father in her mind, *go to sleep.* He is waiting.

"That's hard to do, isn't it? Want some help?" he asks gently.

Maybe he isn't waiting for me, Carrie thinks. *Maybe he just wants to help.* "No," she says, "I think it's easier if I do it myself. You see, it's just this little rubber band I have to get on." But he keeps watching her. He gets into his sleeping bag; he is tucked away, just his eyes open still. Carrie quickly puts the rubber bands in, turns away to take off her shirt, and slips into her own bag, curling away from his eyes and looking up at the gray netting of the tent window. Feeling the warmth of her sleeping bag and hearing that he is still in his, she closes her eyes.

"Goodnight," she says, her eyelids pressed tight.

"Goodnight," Lee says, sounding too awake. Carrie hesitates, then sinks slowly into sleep.

Starting out of dreams, she hears a sound. She hears crickets lulling, but something more: a rustling on the tent floor. *Is he pulling his sleeping bag off? No,* she thinks, murmuring back half asleep, *he is just turning in his sleep.*

Footsteps across the floor. Slowly, as slow as she can so he won't tell she is awake, Carrie tightens her hold on the sleeping bag. Silence except for his creeping. Each of her fingers clasps the bag, she shuts her eyes tight, breathes deeply. *Go away, can't you see I'm asleep?* She forces her breath out slow, heavy, *GO AWAY.*

She smells his sweat. He is kneeling close. Lee pulls gently on her bag. Carrie clenches tighter. Lee laughs. They both know what is happening now.

"Come on, Carrie, come on," he whispers.

She is silent, only concerned with holding the bag tight. She swallows, words come out choked: "I don't want to do anything with you."

He pulls harder on the top of the bag. She grits and holds on. Thinking, she goes inward, internal circles of thought around, around. *I recognize this smile he has, I am too weak to fight him off, but if I could fight him off for long, but he loves me, but he's pulling hard. GO AWAY.* "You see," Carrie says clenching, the words sputtering, "I have many books of experience, many volumes of experience, and I'm not ready for this one yet."

"Huh?" He stops tugging for a moment and laughs. "Did you make that up or read it in a book?" His voice is soft, honestly surprised.

She wants to divert him, send that look out of his eyes. "I just thought of it myself. Have you ever thought of anything like that?" Her braces hurt and he is chuckling and standing up. *Good, he is going away.*

But, no, he grabs the bottom of her sleeping bag, he shakes Carrie out. Naked on the tent floor; it is a battle of smooth hard skin now. She kicks him in the stomach and moves away. "Oh," he says aloud. He knows she is serious, she knows she has hurt him, but he keeps on coming. She struggles, she pushes away. Her brother is sleeping in the other tent outside; maybe she could call him. She could call him, but she doesn't want him to find out she is so naked. The tent walls are heavy. He is excited by this fight, he grabs her by the arms, locking, and she goes limp. It is too much; she knows she is too weak to fight back. Carrie retreats inside herself, closes her eyes, and lets him take her.

He carries her over to his bedding, two sleeping bags unzipped on top of each other. His daughter in his arms, he puts Carrie down softly, a prize, covers her with the bag and lies hot next to her. Kissing her all over, down her belly, down, she cringes.

It happens again the next morning, the next night and the morning after that. In the afternoons Carrie sits on granite boulders watching Lee and Keith dig sewer lines. She sits silent and sullen, hating her father, feeling his acrid sweat staining her skin.

The third day Carrie is sitting on a boulder and Lee climbs up to her, carrying an old pup tent. He holds it up high. "Sew up the holes in this tent and you could sleep in it, if you want." He hands it to her; she smiles and nods. *Maybe he does love me.* Watching him walk away, Carrie sees something hurting in him, stooped in him; she is glad.

Carrie takes the pup tent and it becomes her pride that afternoon, mending it, sewing it, black thread holding in the window's netting firmly. She sets it in a nest of pine trees that night and lies there in her own green gold silk soft sleeping bag, leaving the window open so she can see out into those stars.

MAGGIE HOYAL

"Because I could never talk about what had happened to me, it dominated my life. Then, through my writing, I discovered that I have an intellect that is not stupid but unstretched, a heart which can feel more than pain, a body that once again belongs to me."

Maggie Hoyal was born in Florida on January 15, 1952. Her mother was a registered nurse; her father a member of the local pipe fitters union and an ex-pilot in the air force. Her parents' marriage was one of many separations and reconciliations. Maggie's father began molesting her at the age of nine months and continued to do so until she ran away from home at sixteen. "I remember walking away from the room my father rented," she writes, "feeling the most complete freedom of my life."

For the next five or six years, Maggie repressed all thoughts and feelings about the past. "I did not think at the time that I was running away from memories," she explains. "I had simply put the past out of my mind altogether. At age twenty-two, I remember thinking I had never heard the sound of my own voice above a normal speaking tone. I had never yelled, never screamed, never felt anger or expressed it. I began to wonder why."

At this point Maggie moved to California and became part of a women's writing workshop, where she found, in her words, "one other person who wanted to listen, and after listening, was angry for me." As she began writing, she learned to respect herself for the first time because she had survived. She also began to regard herself with compassionate humor.

When she finished "These Are the Things I Remember," she felt triumphant; it was the first writing she had ever completed. It changed her life. She no longer needed to fail. The story was originally published in P'an Ku, a college literary magazine. "I would like women to realize that we cannot afford a low self-concept because it makes us victims," she states. "We as women do not have to fight our way into a place in this world, nor do we have to beg for one. We are a part of the world to the extent and limit of our own imaginations. Without us, the world is unbalanced and dangerous."

These Are the Things I Remember

I remember the train. The thick metal plate ran even with the level of my chin. My mother's hand pulling me up that first step and the steam blasting from under like a dragon's breath. I sat next to my brother and kept looking across at mother's face, her expression of troubled annoyance. I wondered why she didn't feel it, the excitement of the train.

"Mama, the train."

She looked at her watch and said, "Yes, I know the train is always late."

"But, mama—"

"Quiet down. When you get used to it, the train won't seem like anything, just a train."

It was a warm Florida night, but we stood there in our pajamas shivering in a little line like dominoes. Dickie was first because he was the oldest. Daddy had gone to find the stick. The stick was a piece of pinewood twenty-one inches long and two and a half, three inches wide. "Stick" was the only name it ever had.

I was so scared my teeth chattered when I tried to talk.

"You think he'll hit us real hard?" I said.

"Shoot, he can't hit that hard," Dickie said.

"Only hard enough to kill us," Bobbie put in.

"Why, he don't hit any harder than a fly shits," Dickie said.

"Dickie!" I cried, my mouth hanging open.

Bobbie started to giggle way down in his gut. He was holding his stomach and covering his mouth at the same time, trying not to laugh out loud.

"No harder than a fly shits!" Bobbie repeated.

That was all it took. We were gone, laughing till tears came to our eyes. Laughing 'cause we were too scared to do anything else. Laughing just because we knew we shouldn't be. The scareder we got, the harder we laughed.

Then we heard footsteps coming from the next room. Angry thudding sounds. My father's red face appeared in the doorway and he was swinging Stick at his side.

"So you think it's funny, do you? We'll just see how funny you think this is. Get over here, Dickie."

I plugged my fist into my mouth, but I couldn't stop the giggling sound.

"Pull down your pants and bend over the bed."

Dickie had stopped laughing, but he didn't look afraid. I heard the smack of the hard board on flesh and went silent. Dickie didn't make a sound. His face had a flat quality now, like he was pressed in upon himself. The only sound was the smack of Stick as it hit. Daddy was getting angrier and I could tell he wouldn't let it go until Dickie cried, and I knew Dickie'd never do that. It seemed like it was going to just go on like that forever. Then I heard the crack of wood as Stick splintered in two pieces. One part hit the wall over our heads with a bang and made me jump. The other side hit the floor.

Then everything was silent.

There was a dim light shining just above the sofa on a wooden shelf and mother was reading us stories from the red book. I know it must have been up north on one of our visits to grandma because mama never read when daddy was around, and because of the wood and the winter light as it faded into a later and later hour. My brothers snuggled close to her on either side and I was propped up on the arm. My head moved in and out of the circle of their warmth as each time the page was turned I would be drawn in to see the new and wondrous picture. Sometimes I would close my eyes and listen to the sound of the words, willing them not to stop. It became hard to hold my head up. I edged off the worn sofa arm into a tiny corner next to my brother and lay my head back against its softness.

"You can't sit here," Bobbie said as he pushed me. "It's my place."

Mother looked at me as if she were far away looking at another girl in another time. Her eyes were very sad. She moved her hand over my brother's arm. "There's room for you, baby," she said, and then, remembering my brothers, she added, "There's room for all of you."

She pulled me beside her and wrapped her arm around my shoulders as she continued reading, her arm resting there as if forgotten.

We were asleep when it started. It was mama's voice that woke me up. I had never heard it sound like that, hard and biting.

"It won't work this time," she said.

"Don't you say that," daddy said.

"I told you, Dick, if it happened again I was going to leave you."

"That's your damn English talking."

"It's not right what you do to her!"

I sucked in my breath. What was mama saying?

"She didn't wake up. She doesn't even have to know it happened," he said.

"For God's sake, you promised to stop."

"I will, I will. Just say you won't leave me."

"There is something wrong with you, Dick. It's not safe for the children to be—"

It was then that he struck her, cutting off the words with a hard slap. "You're never taking my kids away from me."

I wanted this not to be happening. I got out of bed and walked soundlessly to the door. I tried to stop shaking. When I looked through the cracked opening into the living room, I could see mama holding the side of her face and tears coming down.

He grabbed her arm and dragged her into the bathroom and threw her to the floor. "No one's ever taking my kids. I'll see 'em dead first."

That was when mama screamed and I started out the door and halfway into the living room. His back was to me, but I could see him put his hands around her throat and squeeze. I tried to scream, but the sound wouldn't come out of my throat. When he stood up, mama was lying in a limp heap upon the bathroom floor. He just stood there looking down at her.

I thought she was dead. He brought his arms up and started rubbing his hands like they were tired. It scared me. I thought any minute he was going to turn on me, so I ran softly into the bedroom and closed the door back the way it was.

If my brothers were awake, they never said so. I never talked about it to anyone.

One morning mama was gone. We kept waiting for her to come home. But when daddy came in from work that night, he brought

a lady with him and he told us mama was gone for good and this
was our new mama. That night I was alone in my small bed on
the far side of the room. My brothers slept in the army bunk beds
that rested against the other wall. The lady that was not our
mother had tucked us in and kissed our cheeks. Before the light
snapped off, I noticed she had wrong-colored hair, and afterward
there was only the silence of the house, empty of mother.

I cried quietly at first, not wanting my brothers to hear, but
then it took over, the crying, and I didn't care anymore. I hoped
the darkness would hide me, and the silence. Muffled footsteps
came into the room and the light ruined my face, exposed it,
swollen-eyed and smeared with tears that wouldn't stop even
then.

"Are you okay, honey?" the lady that was not our mother
asked.

Dickie pushed himself up on an elbow and brushed the hair out
of his eyes. "Aw, she's just crying about our mother. Don't worry
about her. We like you fine."

"Yeah, we think you're prettier, too," Bobbie stuck in, "and
anyway she's just bein' a baby."

"You miss your mama, honey, is that it?"

I cut off the woman's words, pushed them away in my mind
and kept repeating over and over my brother's words.

"You're a baby, you're a baby."

I knew if I kept thinking on those words I could stop crying. I
could push the pain behind the anger and hide it there until the
lady was gone and it was safe again in the darkness.

"That's right. See, you've stopped crying like a good girl. You
go on back to sleep now."

When the light went off, I pushed my face hard into the pillow
and let the sob come, but this time there was no sound, just the
wetness growing in a circle around my face.

I don't remember the day mother came back, I only know that something ended between us.

I came to her only because there was no one else. I was eight years old, but I remember, even in that first vision of St. Lucia, walking across the island sand, which shone white even in the darkness that was undisturbed by cities. I remember thinking how beautiful the world was. The wind sweeping in from the ocean. I remember thinking nothing ugly could happen here.

It was the first motel built on the island, and dad had been the foreman on the job. Instead of the promised bonus for finishing the job early, we were all guests in the motel.

We were on our way to supper at the motel dining room. It was the first time we had to dress in our best clothes before we could go and eat. Mom and dad went first, quietly talking, my brothers following behind like two hungry dogs at their heels. I was walking behind the others, not wanting to ruin the beauty, the sounds of the night, with words. I saw the shadow first as it crossed mine in the white sand—the dark husk of a man before me in the sand—and I jumped. I had been warned about the native men, but then I realized it was only dad.

He began to speak in hushed, urgent tones. "It will be different here," he said.

"What?"

"There won't be anyone to disturb us. . . . Oh, don't pretend," he continued. "You know what I'm talking about."

It hit me, what he meant. I had thought it was over. I had thought it couldn't happen here. I'd put it out of my mind as if it had never happened at all. Him hanging on my door when I got undressed at night, the back-door touching whenever mom was at work. Whenever no one was there to go to, to stop him. I couldn't think of anything to say. I felt tired, and all the beauty of the island was defeated in that moment. Now it was a dangerous place, isolated and lawless.

"Don't worry. I'll take care of your mother so she'll never know."

"But—"

"Don't worry. I'll take care of everything."

He walked away then.

Even if I had thought of anything to say, it was too late.

A few days later, when mother was shopping and the boys were scouting out the island, it began. I heard it in his voice when he called my name. I didn't answer, but he knew I was in my room. After calling a second time, he became angry and yelled for me to come.

I still didn't move.

He walked into my room, but instead of being angry like I thought he would be, he was smiling.

"Take down your pants," he said.

"What'd I do?" I said.

He was still smiling, as if he were in a dream.

"Why?" I answered in a small voice.

He moved toward me.

"It's wrong," I said.

"Your damn mother and her Victorian morals. There's no place for them here. I'm not going to let you turn out cold like your mother."

"I'll tell her."

He grabbed my arms and held them to my sides. His hand slipped down between my legs. His voice was soothing then. He didn't notice that I struggled.

I could feel myself against his hand. I wanted to cry, but I couldn't. I couldn't do anything. I felt the same as when I tried to jump across a mud flat next to a creek and landed short. I started sinking in, and when I pulled at one foot, the other went in deeper. That's what it felt like, sinking.

He pulled his hand out of my pants and spit on his fingers and rubbed them together. He didn't even seem aware of me. The sound of his spitting made me sick. Then he put his hand back down my pants and started to say something in that singsong voice he used.

The front screen door slammed and his hand ripped out of my pants like it was burned. Then he turned on me and whispered harshly, "Don't you say anything to your mother ever. If you do, you'll be sorrier than you've ever been in your life."

I made the bathroom and locked the door. Something that always made my father angry. He used to tease me mean about it, saying I was a prude, like it was something stupid to be. I pulled my pants down and took soap and water and washed off the spit. When I came out, my brothers were there eating sandwiches. The day went on like nothing had ever happened.

At dinner, mom said, "You're awfully quiet, you sick?"

I just shook my head and looked down at my plate. She got up and came over to feel my head.

"You don't feel warm, but you'd better get to bed early just the same."

"Don't baby the girl, she's probably just sulking."

"Just the same, Dick, she don't look right. It wouldn't hurt to be careful."

"There's not a damn thing wrong with her."

"You're probably right."

"Damn right I'm right. You might be a smart little RN and gone to college, but don't know half of nothing."

"I'm sorry, I didn't mean anything."

"Why, your mother didn't even know how to cook when I married her. I had to teach her. And she sure didn't know anything about being a mother, or a woman, for that matter! Still don't know how to be."

"I been trying, Dick."

"Well, just don't try and tell me I don't know what I'm talking about."

My mother nodded silently and got up to start the dishes.

When dad went off to work the next day, I tried to get my mother alone. Her friends were visiting from the other side of the island, and she made coffee and served little cakes.

I had always been quiet; it was hard for me to talk when other people were around, and I knew that mom would be annoyed at being disturbed.

"Mom, I have to talk to you," I said.

The other people in the room stopped talking and looked at me.

"Oh, is that your daughter?" one woman said. "Why, she looks just like you."

I remember grimacing.

"What do you want?" mom said.

"I want to talk to you alone."

"Oh, this is silly. Excuse me, Marsha, I'll be back in a minute."

When we got in the room, she turned to me impatiently and said, "What's wrong, Molly, are you sick?"

"No . . ."

When anyone looked upset, that was the first thing my mother asked. She always looked disappointed when it wasn't that one thing she knew how to fix.

"Then what is it? You interrupted our guests."

"It's about dad. He's . . . he's doing things."

"What things?"

"He makes me let him look at me and . . . he touches me."

"Where? Where does he touch you?"

All I could do was look down in embarrassment.

"It's wrong, isn't it?" I said. "It's wrong what he does."

Mother didn't answer.

"Doesn't it say it's wrong to do that in the Bible? Doesn't it?"

"Yes, yes, of course it does."

"Will you make him stop?"

I heard the sound of laughter coming from the other room. Mother heard it, too. I could hear it in her voice, I could see it in the way her eyes were already darting back and forth toward the door. It was as if my mother were caught and wanted to get away. Back to the safety of polite conversation and meaningless laughter.

"Now listen, I have to go, they will be wondering, but I'll talk to your father and none of this will ever happen again." As she started to leave the room, she turned back, her face directed toward me but not looking at my eyes. "If it does, you let me know."

I stood alone in the room, staring at the door as it closed after her.

When I was fourteen, my parents were divorced and I went with my father and my brother Bob. We were living at the Pine Grove Apartments in Miami. My brother was gone a lot because he was dating a girl my father didn't like. I didn't hear from my mother, but I knew about where it was she lived.

I was going to school and taking care of all the household chores—washing, shopping, and cooking. It was awkward because I had so much to do and I was so afraid to make a mistake. My father thought everything should be perfect. I remember I had just brought the groceries in. I walked to the store and carried the two large bags the five blocks back home. I had just set them down on the counter and collapsed into a chair when my father came barging through the door.

"What are you doing on your butt? The groceries aren't even put away."

I jumped up and headed toward the kitchen.

"Hurry up and make dinner, I'm hungry—no, fix me a drink first."

There was something about his voice that worried me. It was the old feeling of something crawling up the back of my neck.

"You know those clothes you bought last week?"

The question took me by surprise and I didn't answer right away.

"You know who bought those clothes? Me! You just show the little card and think everything is for free. It's not free, I pay for it. And now you have to pay for it."

I hadn't had new clothes in three years and it was dad who'd said I couldn't go around looking the way I did. "I don't want no ragamuffin for a daughter. Take the card and plan to spend about a hundred dollars."

By the time I got through the underwear and the bras and a few skirts and blouses, that was it. I was amazed at how fast it went.

"Now you have to pay for it," he said. "That was the deal."

Dad had said I would be happier I had chose him 'cause he would make me be something, not like mother. She was ruining Dickie by taking him away from discipline, spoiling him.

"He'll be just like all my brothers and sisters, failures. Not one of 'em any good except maybe Pauline, but she's more like a man than a woman should be."

That was the worst thing anyone could be when we were growing up. A failure.

I guess that's some of the reason I went with dad. It didn't seem like there was a choice. Mom never contradicted him about it, and though dad was strict, nothing ugly had happened in several years and I thought that was over. Mom and I were always at odds then and the only thing I felt from her besides annoyance was a void. That frightened me even more than dad did. With dad, at least I felt it mattered that I existed.

But it was like that. Spaces of years where the molesting seemed like a bad nightmare that had happened once to someone else—and then, out of nowhere, there it was.

"What do you mean, pay for it? I don't have any money. Anyway, you told me to buy the clothes. It was your idea."

"Don't talk stupid. Fix me another drink."

I was afraid and confused.

But then dad sat back and smiled at me like he was proud of me all of a sudden. "You know, I'm going to take you and Bob back with me to St. Lucia. Things could be good there. I'll get my flying license back again, like when I was an officer in the air force, and we'll start our own business. Just the real Muellers— Dickie won't get nothing. He don't deserve to be a Mueller.

"And you—why, you won't even know yourself. Molly, you'll be an independent woman, not like your mother. You'll be free. I'm going to teach you how to fly better than any man, and just you and me we'll make a damn good business jockeying tourists back and forth between the islands. Bob, he'll do all the paper work and keep things going right while we fly our heads off."

It sounded like a dream. I thought about how it would be, flying all alone sometimes, just me and—

"But we have to get this other stuff out of the way first."

"What other stuff?"

"You and me. We have to go through with it and get to the other side. You're getting older now and you know other boys. Maybe some of those rich tourists are going to start dating you. You can't keep feeling the way you do about me. I'm your father, and when you meet some special boy, then you'll find you come to love him like you think you love me now. I know you won't think so now, but someday this will just be a memory in the past."

I felt like I was sinking. I leaned on the counter and tried to think the thing out.

My God. He thinks I want to . . . Jesus. He thinks it's me that . . .

It was the first time I really realized he was sick. Before, I had just pushed it all out of my mind. Now I had to face it, to face him. I kept thinking I had to trust myself now. I wondered what he would do if I told him he made me sick.

I thought about it, fucking him. My mind just couldn't keep hold of it. I wondered if I could take that. Then I thought about him. What would it do to him if I told him what I really thought. Would he go crazy? Was he crazy?

The argument wove in and out—first the threat, *you owe me;* and then what was worse, the pleading: *I'm your father, trust me, trust me.* And then, what if I told him he was insane?

I had to decide.

I was so tired of it drilling at me like a tedious argument that would never, never end. I thought, If I do it, maybe then it will be over with for good. He will finally have what he wants and leave me alone.

I thought, Okay, you motherfucker, I'll trust you once.

Maybe I was just tired of fighting, tired of having no one to go to. Tired of wondering who was right. My father had told me that mom already knew everything, and that my brothers knew about it, too.

When I was twelve, Bob had caught me packing to run away and he just laughed at me. "You run away? You don't have it in you. What do you want to go for anyway?"

I had started to cry. I told him about dad. What had been going on. He knew what I meant.

"I have to run away, Bob."

"No, you don't want to go and do that," he said. "Dad must know what he's doing, he's our father—he knows what's best."

After that, I knew there would never be any help from Bob.

My father interrupted my thoughts for the millionth time. "Well . . . ?"

"All right, all right, I'll do it. But I have my period now."

Then there was no pretense about teaching me or doing what was good for me.

"When is it going to be over?"

"I don't know," I said sharply.

It was the longest period I ever had, but finally even I knew that it wouldn't work for much longer.

It was in the middle of the afternoon when dad drew the line.

"Now," he said.

"But—"

"I don't believe that period shit. If you still have it, show me your pad."

"Listen, forget it. I never wanted to do it anyway. You keep pushing it and pushing it."

"See? I knew you were lying."

"I wasn't lying. I had my period."

"I knew it, you said 'had.' See? You said 'I *had* my period.' You can't fool me, I knew you were lying. I was just waiting for you to own up to it yourself."

I was trapped. My period had been over for five days. I was caught in a lie that, no matter how inconsequential, seemed to discredit anything I had to say. I couldn't seem to win.

"I know you better than you know yourself, that's why I know what's best for you better than you do, or ever will, for that matter.

"Now," he said, "take off your clothes."

"In the middle of the day? What about Bob?"

"Bob won't be home till later. He's busy, and anyway you don't have to worry about him. Hurry up."

I stood there. My toes seemed to try to crawl under the terrazzo floor. I was looking at the cold white bed. The room was filled with icy air and white light shifting through the pale green curtains. I wanted to say something. I wanted to say no.

"I don't want to," I said.

"That's over with now. It's been decided." His voice was threatening now, dangerous.

"I have to go."

"Go then, but make it short."

My legs were trembling. I looked into the bathroom mirror and laughed softly into it, at the lovely creature, the scared girl, staring out at me.

I had never even gone on a date. I looked like I was ready to
attend my first party.

"Come on, get done and get out of there."

"Coming," I yelled back. Even here he won't leave me alone, I
thought bitterly.

I thought of locking the door.

There was no lock.

Damned cheap apartments, they can't even afford privacy for
the john door. Can't even lock the door on your father when he's
crazy and you're scared.

I thought of Bob. A glint of hope that maybe he would come.
At the next moment, the door would open and put a stop to the
whole miserable thing. Then I laughed again into the mirror, No,
no pretending, not now. No, dad was right, Bob was busy. He
wouldn't be back till it was too late to matter.

Then I thought I would break down, and the tears stung in my
eyes. Bob, how could you leave me here with this crazy man, who
doesn't even know what crazy is?

"I'm coming in there to get you if you don't get out of there
soon."

I started taking off my blouse, not wanting to undress in front
of him. After all this time, my breasts were growing. How I hated
them in that moment. My body was late at doing everything. I
had thought my breasts would never grow, and now the joy of it,
of becoming a woman, was twisted and stolen from me.

"No!" I screamed, but the words never left my mouth.

I took off my skirt and panties. My belly was brown and
smooth. I hadn't put on any lazy fat yet. My clothes fell to the
floor. I should fold them, I thought, and then wanted to cry again.
They were the new clothes I had just bought. They were carelessly pretty in the tight, short style of Miami in the Sixties. City of
light. Artificial city where the sun never touches the cold irony of
its people, drifting from air-conditioned apartments to neon bars.

I touched the cold sheets. His touch was cold, too, his sloppy groping gestures hidden under the sheets. The touch of his hanging belly on top of mine. The smell of Old Spice and Canadian Club breathing down on me from his sloppy open mouth. He wasn't drunk. He was never drunk, just undignified. He felt my cunt with his fingers and then, like a doctor prescribing a medicine, he said, "We'll just get some baby oil and then it won't hurt at all. You're lucky I am doing this for you the first time and not some punk in the back seat of a car."

I was beyond thinking and feeling then.

I remember the putrid smell of baby oil and the cold wet oil dripping from my thighs. I remember saying over and over to myself, It will be over soon, it will be over soon, it will be over . . .

The shock of the searing pain so deep inside me, I knew no one had a right to that. I pulled away, furiously struggling to get free. I screamed. He looked at me with contempt.

"It doesn't hurt that much. I used the baby oil so I know."

It was then that I started screaming, "No, *get off me! Get off me!*"

He seemed shocked. "Take it easy now. Well, maybe it does hurt the first time a little. Okay, calm down, okay."

His body slid across me like a great lumpy slug.

I closed my eyes for a second to squeeze the tears back.

He went to touch me, but I jerked away.

I crawled from the bed, my cunt aching like it had been sliced open. I walked slowly to the bathroom, a trickle of blood running in a thin, delicate line down my thigh.

YARROW MORGAN

"The earliest time I can remember being molested was when I was three to five months old."

Yarrow Morgan was born in 1947 in Beresford, South Dakota. She was molested by her father and mother from infancy until she was seven or eight years old, and by a brother in early childhood. When she was about four, Yarrow told her mother about the sexual abuse by her father. Her mother became enraged:

"'Don't you ever say that about your father again!' she screamed, and began to strangle me. I lost consciousness. When I came to, she told me to forget all about what had happened. Her face was very angry and very frightened. She knew I was telling the truth. I did forget—both that incident and my father's molesting me."

Yarrow sees promiscuity, drug abuse, isolation, difficulty in trusting, and picking abusive sexual partners as some of the harmful consequences of her abuse. "My healing began with my simultaneous decisions to accept myself as a lesbian and to enter therapy," she writes. She worked for five years with a therapist primarily on incest issues, and went through a chemical-dependency program for women that emphasized integrated sexuality as crucial to dealing with alcohol and drug issues.

Yarrow is a lesbian writer, a healer, and a produce worker living in Minneapolis, Minnesota. "Remember," excerpted here, was published in the magazine Sinister Wisdom and in an anthology that Yarrow and Toni McNaron edited entitled Voices in the Night: Women Speaking About Incest, published June 1982 by Cleis Press.

from **Remember**

"Be quiet. Go to sleep now.
Mommy and Daddy are here."

Three-year-old girl child
lay in her bed,
drowsy and safe
awake not asleep.
She saw a pink and purple
wormlike thing above her body.
It did not touch her, no,
it pulsed in the air.
It was going to touch her.
Her screaming woke the house.
Woke her mommy who listened
and said, "It's not real,
it's not real; go back to sleep,
it's not real; it didn't happen."

"You were such a good baby, so quiet,
you could just sit still for hours!
You never cried."

She lay in her crib,
infant eyes open, unfocused—
only things very close really seen.
Like the crib bars,
long and square and golden.
Her breathing sucks in and out
like curling ocean waves,
rolling up in swirls of pleasure
from belly to lips and back down again.

The space about her body seems infinite;
full of huge beings, strange smells,
and feelings vibrate as the dust-motes
in the air, that catch her eyes
and turn golden.
A being she knows comes close.
He touches her
and she is enveloped in safety.
He takes off her clothes
and she kicks her feet in the air laughing.
He laughs and tickles her.
Then he places upon her
the long purple-pink globe of flesh
that has a life of its own.
It covers her body
from chest down to between her legs,
which are now forced back
and up into the air.
Her flesh curls inside her—
away from both him and herself.
She does not cry out.
She does not let herself know
any of the feelings
the vast air now swirls with.

Blank it out.
Don't let yourself know it's real.
If it's real, you're crazy; blank it out.
Knowledge is powerlessness.
Blank it out.
Knowledge is pain.
Blank it out.
Mother to daughter;
blank it out.

Teach us to numb ourselves,
teach us not to feel.

The memory does not come easy;
it comes with screams that will not stop,
it comes with tears and terror,
it comes with shame that I felt this,
shame that I feel this.
The memory does not come easy;
I tell you because I know,
I tell you because I will not be silent,
I tell you because I will not be silenced.

JEAN MONROE

"In the story I have a protective feeling for my father, which is, of course, screwy as hell."

Jean Monroe (a pseudonym) was born in the early Forties. Twenty-six years after her father stopped abusing her, she wrote "California Daughter/1950." The complete version was published in Aphra *magazine in 1976 and is listed in the category "Most Distinctive Stories" in* Martha Foley's Best Stories *the same year.*

Almost thirty years after the abuse, Jean still expressed conflicting feelings. "I have a great fear of the story," she writes. "My relationship with my parents is very fine these days, and I fear that someday, sometime, they will come across it. I still want to protect them."

She continues: "It is all so complex and I distrust, I guess, my own accounting of it. For instance, I have often maintained that I was not very hurt by the experience.... As an adult I've always been very happy sexually. Somehow I got an affirmative sense of my own personal sexual power from my father." But she quickly adds: "Make no mistake about this. I DID NOT ENJOY IT!"

"Betrayal is a basic theme in my life," she continues. "I am sure it is a hurt that goes back to my father. What a terrible betrayal. My father is a fine man who prides himself on his high moral principles. How he could have betrayed a child, his child, is still overwhelming to me."

From California Daughter / 1950

The children are in their bedroom, far away, but their voices, their laughter falls here through the living room. I wish I were with them.

Gently he asks me if I would mind unbuttoning my pajama top. Of course not, I assure him, and quickly do it. A small figure scurries across the hall entrance and he yells, "I told you to stay in the bedroom! Your sister and I ʌre talking. Now get back in there."

They embarrass me. The brown keeps growing in ever-widening circles and the nipples stick out grotesquely when they are exposed to the air. I don't know why he likes them. Someday they'll be big enough for a brassiere.

"Can I touch them?" daddy asks me.

I am shaking my head yes before he finishes the question. His fingers, wrinkled and dark on my white skin, delicately trace the round widening brown circle and the nipple sticks out more. His fingers so lightly like whispering move out on the little mound and slowly down and over. He cups them. He pulls the nipple.

"They are very pretty, honey. You are growing up to be a woman."

The living room is silent except for his breathing. The brother and sister are playing in the bedroom. Daddy is in his armchair and I am on the hassock facing him. The lamp shines above us and onto my bare chest. His eyes are green and I see myself in them, tiny and doubled. I pray to Jesus that soon he'll tell me that I can go. I wish I were playing with the children. We are careful not to let them see.

He moves in the chair. He laughs a little and in a shifting motion with his left hand pushes against his pants. The strange look on his face makes me want to assure him that it's okay. Don't be afraid, daddy, it's okay with me.

I can hear and see and feel his breathing. His eyes are boring into my bare breasts. "Breasts" is a word that is hard for me to say. I wish they were pretty for you, daddy. They seem like sores swelling and when I look down at them I don't understand. I do nothing and they keep swelling.

"Don't ever tell anyone, baby. They wouldn't understand. This is strictly between us, okay?"

He bends his face close to them and I smell the hair oil on his large head, his hair wavy and red-brown, the lashes of his eyes caught in the light. You don't have to worry, daddy, I'll never tell. His hot breath stirs the nipple and his fingers seem larger than my ribs.

Suddenly the bedroom door bangs open and the children come running down the hallway. Daddy hastily closes my top and slides back in his chair. When they come into the room, he is cold to them, but I am relieved, thankful they have come.

"What are you playing?" My voice sounds strange, the words forced.

"Hide-and-seek! You're it!" she yells, hitting me and running.

I jump up and run with them, furtively buttoning my pajamas. But I feel foolish. I'm nine years old and too big to be playing their games. My stomach feels funny. I know this is only acting.

* * *

Darkness outside we move through, watching, noses against cold steamy windows. We go to see mama. Lights flicker in the black; our car is filled with us, our warm bodies, and daddy's, and our breathing. The children sit at the windows in the back, and I sit in the mother's seat. The passing cars think I am the mother. On Friday nights we always go to the Pike in Long Beach and buy shrimp. We walk down the central mall to see the strange sights, a mummified hung cowboy, dancing chickens, tattoo parlors, sailors watching naked-girl movies in the machines, fat ladies without teeth calling to us to play the games.

"Hey, babe!" they cackle after daddy, and he laughs. But we are too broke to play. Rhythmic screams like a song from the giant roller coaster fling out over the night ocean, a man sits atop a high pole for months, breaking a record. It's in the newspapers. We buy the shrimp and french fries and drive eating to the tuberculosis sanatorium on Signal Hill. Daddy drives the car across the dark dead lawn, between the groaning oil wells, black long-nosed monsters, to her window. He leaves us in the car. I see him tapping the window, and after a while she lifts the window and I see her dark form. Someday she'll come home.

* * *

I go to the garage to get my bike and he is there, working in his lighted corner. I know I am trapped.

"Honey, come back here a minute."

I slide between him and the car fender and when he asks I lift my T-shirt. He touches them and I smile when he looks at my face. I must show him it is all right with me. But I don't like it. They are larger and more embarrassing, cold puckering the skin around the nipples. He is funny, breathless and giggly, different from his usual stern self. But it's not hurting me, and if I object, it will hurt him. He would see then that I know it is wrong. I couldn't bear for him to think that. Poor daddy. It's all right. The tools hang on the boards of the tar-papered garage, Marilyn Monroe curls down pink and naked from the calendar.

"Remember," he says, his huge finger over and over the protruding nipple, "remember, this is just between you and me. Don't tell anyone. Especially mama."

He likes to take his thing out of his pants for me to look at it. He seems to love it. "Isn't it nice?" It's ugly, purple, veined, worse than varicosed legs. He's so interested in it, I pretend it's nice.

It isn't something that I dwell on, yet I know when it's coming and I seek ways to avoid him. When I'm cooking dinner and he's due home from work, I get the children to play on the kitchen floor. I try hard to act oblivious so that he won't understand my understanding. He loves me, he loves me; somewhere I understand his need.

Mama comes home from the hospital. My brother and I are standing at the foot of the neighbor's driveway, watching our friends playing in the yard, when our sister comes down the street shouting. There's a surprise for us at home. When we get there, it is mama. Standing in the living room with her back to the heater, she is smiling at us, her hands folded behind her. The whiteness of her skin from lack of sun is astonishing.

We sense immediately that we must stay back, something in her stern quietness. It is the first thing that is said.

"Mama came home sooner than the doctors wanted her to. She left without permission because she knew she would die there. She's come home to get well, but you must not get near her."

She remains in bed for a while, only getting up to wash her own dishes that must be kept separate. The coffee cup with the smudge of lipstick, the glass, the utensils, the plate, all take on the forbidden quality of mama. The word "germs" is used often and I know that they are in her body. But her body and, most important, her mind are strong, stronger than the doctors think. Gradually she is up more. If you think you are well, she says, then you will be. If you think you are dying, then you will die.

My chores grow less as she becomes our normal mother again. In a year I have forgotten how to cook and iron and I wonder how I was able to do it before. She is strong, her body and ways serious and different, it seems, from other mothers, other people. She rarely laughs and she has no other interests than us. Her body is voiceless, still, surer than all words and gestures, all diseases, and always there. I step out, but she is there to come back to. Her body isn't like the one on the calendar, it doesn't lilt in the S curve, and she would never smile in that way. Naked, it's almost ugly. Her stomach is large, her thighs and breasts hang like heavy sacks, but I come to understand that it is the body of a mother, and the other, that of a girl.

* * *

As she becomes well, daddy grows colder, a brooding dark figure moving heavily through the house. As always, she explains him to us: He's unhappy in his work. He works long hours at a job he hates in order to feed us and take care of us. He hates it, but he does it for us. He's young. He could be many things. Many men couldn't do it; they'd leave. Your father will never run away. He loves us.

I avoid his eyes. He is angry. He stays away some nights and I hear my mother awake, waiting for him. He seems mad at me, yells, accuses me of things I don't understand, and I become mad, too. You are just like him, she says then, over and over. You are just like him. Proud. You feel deeply for others, but you are proud. Southern pride. False pride. I am told through it all that it's because he loves me. He argues with you because he loves you. You are his favorite child; you're just like him. He hugs me when he comes home from work, pressing me hard against his hard penis, my tender breasts mashed up against his chest, his breath smelling of beer. He was jealous of you when you were born. You took so much of me from him. Now he's becoming jealous of your growing up, growing away from him, of your finding a boyfriend, and eventually a husband. He wants you to love only him. You're a beautiful girl, it worries him sick.

I watch him walking toward us to the car, across a room, in Long Beach where I was born, in downtown Los Angeles, in the

mountains, on the beach working, talking, and always his hand
moves down and touches his penis as if to make sure that it's
there. It's the most important part of him, maybe the only thing
that makes him happy. Handsome. A sad handsome boy-man.
Will I find a husband as perfect? Red-brown curls, the heavy-
lidded eyes that are my eyes.

* * *

I hate it most in the winter when the air is cold and shrivels the
skin. I'm embarrassed. But he says they are beautiful. Never tell,
honey. I love you. I never will, daddy, I promise. They are getting
so big. You are beautiful.

I never miss Sunday school. They press pictures on felt of burning hell and say that if your parents are at home reading the
Sunday paper, or sleeping, this is where they will go. I grow to
know Jesus as myself, and I pray to God the Father, but I know, I
know my parents aren't going to hell. They are good, they are
perfect. I know that Jesus knows them. Forgives them. I pray long
into the night. I pray for others, for the neighbors; I explain to
Jesus their ways; I seem to understand that all their sad and sinful
ways are because they want to be loved. I know it's okay. I pray
that daddy won't ever feel guilty for what he does to me. It's all
right, Jesus, it is really all right. I pray for all the children and
miners and the dead bodies of my ancestors, buried in the South. I
pray for the scared soldiers in Korea. Hours in the dark bed trying
to picture them there, to be with them on the cold, snowy battle-
fields, hiding in the trenches. I pray for some kind of solution to
my father's hated job. Douglas Aircraft plant. The hated foreman.

I understand others, but I seem to lose myself. The inside more
real than the outside. I can't see myself. Lessons, lectures, what
one must do. You must be careful with your reputation. They

write in your school record anything suspicious about your character and you can never escape it. I feel eyes on me, expectant. They are waiting to see what kind of girl you will turn into once your period starts. Good girl or bad? I watch the ways the others hold their bodies, move their mouths, walk, absorbing their mannerisms. I don't know how to be in the world. I can't see what I look like. It is said that I am introverted, and I find comfort in the word. At last mama buys me a brassiere. The sixth-grade boys, all a head shorter than I, pop the elastic on my back. I worry about my record and scream at them. The sudden hysteria shocks me.

* * *

I am walking to the corner market on Industrial, a long block through an empty field, sidewalks littered with broken glass and debris. When I reach the new bachelor apartments across the street from the church, I see a man standing in his open doorway. His pants are down and he is twirling his penis in the dark pubic hair. His face seems aglow and he watches me as I walk, as I walk, trying not to seem alarmed, for I'm not really, trying to act as if I don't see him. The sun glitters in the broken glass. Returning from the market, I walk on the church side, past the tent where Billy Graham hollers and screams every night, and again, he is there, holding it, rubbing it, pumping it up and down, gesturing to me. Smiling.

Every day I go to the store to get the bread. Sometimes I tell my mother of the incidents. I tell her of the two older men who inched their car along beside me as I walked. "C'mon, honey, get in. We have some candy for you." That breathless, giggly mansound. I tell her of them because I was really afraid. But the man in the doorway would be arrested and I can tell he means me no harm. And the old men in the bushes, the winos who suddenly jump out of hiding to show it to me—Little girl, look!—seem strangely helpless, and though I am frightened and run away, how can I tell on them? And what good would it do? There are so many.

I'm stranded inside the store. Outside in the parking lot, a man is waiting in his car for me. I know it. His glassy eyes on me, his tongue out the way men do when they look at you. He blinked his car lights on my bare legs when I walked in front of it and started opening the door. I ran inside. I don't know what to do. I can't tell the man behind the counter. Can I run fast enough across the intersection to my friend's house? What if I get stopped at the traffic light? What if the gate is locked? What if she's not home? It gets later and later. The sun is going down. The grocery man keeps looking at me. Finally I make the dash. His lights hit me just as I run by; I hear his door open and his voice mumbling. I run harder and harder. The gate is unlocked. She's home. I call my mother to come get me.

My closest friend tells me all the words—fuck and shit, and cunt, and screw, and asshole, and cocksucker, motherfucker. She described her parents fucking at night. *"Not yet, not yet,"* her *mother crying. "Now! Do it now, hurry,"* hurry, hurry *through dark open rooms dark nights fathermotherpumpingmoaning crying. Beatings. I love you . . . I hate you. . . .*
We sleep on the sun roof, black iodiny sea-salt night, ocean thumping hard against the earth and the stars and she is saying, "I want to fuck you, let's do it, something happens to you when you do it." She shows me where she has shaved her first pubic hair, black bristly quarter-inch hairs like my father's when he needs a shave, and she rubs against me all night until it seems I will bleed from the rawness. "Something must happen," she keeps whispering, "something must happen," and the loud ocean and all the world is whispering it with her. Something must happen. Something must happen.

We are jumping rope. I have had my turn and now begin turning the rope for Ronnie. He is a boy who lives six blocks away and he has told everyone that he loves me. I feel very strange. I am falling into the street. I am staring at the sidewalk gutter curb, my body lies against it. My mouth is bleeding, I have fallen into the street, and then daddy is picking me up in his arms and carrying me to the house. Are you okay, baby? I am crying and I see tears in his eyes. Ronnie is left alone on the sidewalk.

I begin fainting often when the blood comes.

The bathroom door is shut and I knock, hoping no one is in there.

"Who is it?" Daddy's voice.

Oh, no, it's coming.

"Please come in, honey."

Trapped, can't go away, I walk in. the room is steamy and hot, the shower curtain only half pulled. I know without looking that he is lying in the water. I want to check my pants. I'm frantic that there is blood on the back of my pants. But now I only wash my hands. My back is to him and I pray to God in heaven that there is no blood on the back of me. I'll die. He is talking. I know it is coming.

He holds his thing and I try hard to ignore it. He forces me to look.

"Oh, baby, look at this," he says giggling. "Have you ever seen how big it can get?"

"Oh, yes," I say, feigning interest. It's ugly, purple, hard veins encircling it, pulsing tight in the sudsy water. He pulls it forward, pushes it down as if it has to be forced, as if it has a will of its own. He is proud of it and I can't hurt his feelings.

"Did you know that it can move by itself?" It bobs in the air above the soapsuds.

"Oh, yes, that's nice, daddy." My words seem inadequate, embarrassed.

"Men and boys will be noticing you soon, honey, and they will want to kiss you and touch you. And if you let them, they'll go too far. It's up to the girl to stop it. The sex drive is strong in men, they can't help what they do. They'll plead and beg for you to let them, but if you weaken and give in, they'll hate you. They'll treat you like dirt. They'll tell each other what they have done, and more. They'll call you a whore. And once your reputation is bad, you'll never be able to escape it. They won't marry you. Men only marry virgins. Your virginity is the most wonderful gift you can give your husband. The sex drive is strong in girls, too. But you must be stronger than it. The wisest thing is to never sit and kiss a boy for any length of time. It will overwhelm you and before you know it, before you can help it, you will have gone too far. And he will be looking for another girl, one who is stronger and a challenge."

Mama talks to me every day when I come home from school. She is usually in the bathtub and I sit on the closed toilet seat and she tells me the facts of life.

I move with my naked body in the mirror. The bathroom is steamy, the last of the bath water gurgles down the drain. I open the window to clear the mist. As it changes from heavy mist to wet tears running down the mirror, I pose and smile and throw my head back. Wetting my lips, I move my hand across my breasts and stomach. I am Marilyn Monroe, my body becomes like hers. I paint my lips red and the change is phenomenal. Just one more year and I can wear lipstick. I rub the towel up and down my back, throwing out my hip, and then kiss my mouth on the wet, the wet red lips.

FUCK

I jump.

FUCK

A gasp coming from my throat.

FUCK

My heart pounding. A grizzly old man's face leers at me from the open window. He slips away. I hear his shuffling footsteps.

The humiliation at my own behavior is greater than any fear and I hurriedly leave the bathroom.

Sitting in the car with mama at Douglas's back parking lot, waiting for daddy to get off work, a boy is walking toward us, coming across the landing field. Watching him. He floats across the black asphalt toward me, softly smiling, his eyes, he walks with clouds behind him, staring at me, I want to say something to him, grab him, the angles of my body seem to move out toward him, a plane is taking off in the far field, but I sit here with my mother and I don't understand what all this is, why I feel so excited and confused, but I sense that she does and I am humiliated. I've already fallen, she knows it of me, slut, as she had always feared, and the boy knows, too, the worst kind of woman.

One day I knock on the bathroom door and mama says to come in. Before I leave, she begins telling me again of the dangers of sex. I stand behind the curtain of the hot bathroom. She reclines in the sudsy water and says, "The sex urge is so strong, honey, that some people can't control themselves. They may do things that they know to be wrong and yet they won't be able to help themselves." Through the opened part of the curtain, I can see her soft and saggy breasts floating in bubbles. "Men will want to touch you on your breasts. Breasts excite men and give them sexual pleasure." I have heard all this before, so many, many times.

"Daddy does that to me."

"What?"

"Daddy does that—touches me there." I'm embarrassed to say "breasts." I'm amazed that I've told her.

There is a silence and then she asks, "When does he do this?"

I tell her, "When we are alone." Then I say, "Please don't tell him I told you. I promised him."

Another silence.

"All right," she says in her gentle voice. "But I want you to tell me if he ever does it again. I'm sure that he never will, but if he does, will you tell me?"

"Yes."

"You can go play now."

I start to leave.

"Honey"—her voice gentle, though strange as when she was first sick—"he couldn't help it."

"I know that."

And I leave, jump off the front porch, skipping the steps, and run all the way to Susan's. I feel greatly relieved and happy because I know that I'll never have the problem again. Mama will take care of it.

R.C.

"I unfolded in my own time, in my own rhythm. If you want it, quietly know this: Be gentle with yourself. It will happen."

When R.C. was four years old, her father began coming to her bed and forcing her to have oral sex with him. He continued to do this until she was eleven years old. She repressed the knowledge of these nightly visits during adolescence and throughout many years of her adult life. "I had no recollection of ever having been molested," she writes. "When incest was mentioned, I remember feeling only great anxiety."

At the age of fifteen, she let her schoolmates know that she was available for sex. "I fucked everybody who wanted me. I told them they could do anything they wanted with me if they would pretend they liked me. They did."

She later married a violently disturbed man who abused her to the extent that she repeatedly miscarried. She divorced him and two subsequent husbands who both battered her. "I approached each man from a place of need," she says. "I gave my 'self'... in return for 'love.'"

During this time, she still had no conscious knowledge of her father's abuse. Then, about six years ago, she participated in a growth group. And finally, she remembered: "A woman was talking about her father. I don't remember now what she was saying, but anxiety permeated my stomach and chest. I curled up into a prenatal position. ... All of a sudden, I knew. I felt like throwing up. I knew."

R.C. is completing a master's degree in counseling and hopes to work with other survivors of incest. She has recently come out as

*a lesbian. "To be a lesbian," she concludes, "is to say I fill myself.
I know who I am, and I like me. I have met and loved my rage,
for in my rage comes power. And I am strong!"*

Remembering Dream

I stroll through a tree-lined meadow. Almost hidden among the
trees squats a house, dark and windowless. Blanketed with cobwebs, it is a relic from another time. I want to flee, but find
myself moving closer.

The terror sickness mounts in my throat, almost gagging me as
I near the heavy rotting door. Cautiously, I push the door open. It
groans and splinters. Fine powder rains down from decaying lin-
tel timbers.

It is so dark that the darkness has substance to it, like tension.
With the meager light filtering through the open door, I recognize filthy brown carpeting, beige walls with grimy paint hanging
in long thick peels. I remember now: I was a child in this house.

In my bedroom I discover an old brass bed. In it, among and
beneath cobwebs, lie two bodies. Dead. Skeletal. One is my
grandmother. Greermar. I don't know the other. I stand at the
bedside missing Greermar. My Greermar. Lonely for her, for the
way she loved me. She loved me no matter what I did. Just because I was me. Nothing asked. Nothing expected. I wonder if
anyone will ever love me like that again and all of a sudden I
desperately long for that love. My eyes move from her figure, and
again notice the other body. I know who it is. Of course. It is me.
It is the me that wants to die. That wants to be dead. Dead like
Greermar is dead. Dead with Greermar.

I carry my dead body gently outside. Out into the sunshine.
There appears an opening in the earth. A grave. I place myself in

the hole. I go back and carry out Greermar. I rest her body against mine. We embrace.

Inside, I reenter that bedroom to clean and paint the walls a sunny yellow and build a window for sunshine and fresh breezes.

Turning a corner, I see a door. I begin to shake, and yet I feel drawn. My hands perspire rivulets and leave their damp prints on the dingy brass doorknob. As the door opens, the beam above the doorway dislodges, crashing diagonally across the threshold. My path is blocked. Insects swarm. Termites, wasps, moths escape from the rotted beam blocking even my view. This room does not want me here. I take a deep breath. Strength shoots through my body and I yell, break through, and rush in. I fall on a staircase, rickety and old. It wants me to fall. It wants me OUT OF THERE! I will not leave. I lie down and crawl on my belly, step by step. Some steps are missing. Others are badly splintered, and it is so dark I cannot see. My head bumps something. It is bright. It's a wreath, brown with age. In the center of the wreath is the decapitated head of my mother.

"Don't look!" she screams at me, blocking my way with her terrifying angry-mother look.

I shoot her back a look of my own and say, "Get out of my way."

She disappears and I am at the bottom of the stairs. High up, there is a tiny window. Almost a slit. I must get up there. I shimmy up the exposed wall studs. I am cut and scratched and the pain adds to my determination. On tiptoes I peer trembling through the slit of a window. I see me, four years old. Thin blondish hair. Little girl face. White pajamas with little blue flowers. My father is crying and telling me to be good. He pulls down my pajama bottoms and tries to put something too big inside my vagina. I think about shitting. How this is almost like shitting. Only it's not coming out of me and it is not quite the right place. I am terrified that my father is crying. I won't mind the hurt if it will make him stop crying. The big thing won't go in, though, and he is still crying. He stops and tells me I must love him. I lie still and he puts that big thing into my mouth. He is holding my nose. I can't breathe. He won't stop and I feel guilty for fighting it. He needs me. My mouth fills with stickiness and I am throwing up all over. My mother comes in and hits me for not getting to the toilet in time.

I shove both hands into the slit window and gently lift out the child, cradling her into my body. Rocking, I sob for her. I sob for me. I sob.

JILL MORGAN

"I now own and control my own body and soul, and I know that no man will ever destroy me."

Born in 1950 in a small town in the Midwest where her parents still live, Jill Morgan (a pseudonym) was sexually abused by her father during most of her childhood in a particularly brutal manner. "I told adults of the horror I was enduring, but NO ONE listened," she writes. "Or they believed that my parents were such pillars of the community that they could not be guilty of the crime. Later, therapists referred to Oedipal fantasies instead of listening to what I was saying."

Writing, therapy, and participation in a support group for incest survivors have helped Jill overcome this abuse. She has moved away from her parents. "We all maintain the lie that child abuse and rape did not occur in our house," she states. Her younger sister knows nothing of how her father threatened Jill with raping this sister, too, if Jill did not comply with his demands. Jill wants to protect her sister from this knowledge as she lives close to their father and idolizes him.

Jill has written articles on incest and molestation and hopes to counsel other survivors of child sexual abuse in the future. She continues to heal, to grow stronger and more confident of her own power. Recently she gave birth to her first healthy child, Joey. "I am doing my best to give my daughter a sense of her own power," she writes. "Joey belongs to Joey. She is mine only to teach and influence."

She concludes, "After twenty-six years of pain, I have found some joy and affirmation in my life, and each day has become worth living."

It Began for Me

It began for me the summer I was four years old. My mother had a small baby to care for and worked nights, so my father bathed me. Often he let his soapy hands slide over my vulva.

He would also call me in from play in order to undress me in the empty house and then, with hurried injunctions not to tell mama, send me out to play again.

When he called this time, he took the dog that loved and protected me and locked him in the kitchen. His hands undressing me this time were harsh and angry; his voice abrupt and vicious. I was frightened and questioned him. With a harsh slap, he silenced me. I was used to abuse in that household but not to his strange behavior.

With no words and no warning, he spread my legs and entered me dry. My scream started the dog barking. I must have passed out, because my next memory is of the sunlit garden through the French doors to my right and the sound of the dog barking frantically in the kitchen. My memories here are sketchy. I really don't even remember the pain yet.

When he was through with me, he dropped me on the floor like a discarded dishrag. Then with belt in hand he began beating me. When the belt stopped its endless rise and fall, he took me in the bedroom, re-dressed me in the same play clothes, and put me into my bed with a strict injunction to stay there. I know that I fell asleep crying and comforted myself with the rag doll I found there.

When I awoke, it was black in the room and I could hear the

hum of voices in the house. I began crying again and apparently that attracted the attention of the rest of the family. Finally my mother opened the door and flicked on the light. When I heard her frantic cry, I looked at her and followed her eyes to my blood-soaked bed. To this day I remember her turning to him where he stood behind her in the doorway and saying, "What have you done to her?"

The next thing I remember is the hospital and the sight of a transfusion dripping into my arm. A man dressed in white and standing over me was asking my mother what had happened to me. She answered that she didn't know; I must have fallen down while playing. The man's voice became rough and angry, startling me into tears. He instantly bent down to me and said with infinite tenderness, "It's all right, little one. We're all going to take good care of you." As I felt a needle ease into my arm on the other side, he was saying, "Somebody did this to her!"

I spent several weeks in that hospital and several people came to ask the same questions over and over again. "How did you get hurt? Who hurt you?" Knowing what would happen if I told the truth, I lied. By this time I was pretty confused as to exactly what had happened to me.

When I was finally released, one of the people who had questioned me drove me home. My parents were both there. I remember the man saying, "We know that somebody in this house broke her pelvis and did all of the internal damage. We can't prove anything, but I'll be watching. If she shows up at any local hospitals, I'll know about it and by God I'll make a case stick against you!"

The next few years were calm except for the abuse that naturally occurred in that house, in which I was no more a victim than any of the other kids. My parents moved often in the next five years. Their moves took us to nine different cities.

The second time was when I was nine years old. I knew that I was alone in the house with him but had forgotten enough of the earlier experience to make me feel relatively safe.

I remember his touching me and my squirming away. He slapped me and threw me on a bed nearby. I tried to get up and run, but he caught me and threw me back. Finally he pulled his belt out of his pants and used it to hold me to the bed. He tied my arms to the headboard. I think we both thought about screaming at the same time, because as I opened my mouth he stuffed a dirty stocking in it to shut me up. When he was through, he got up and left. I must have passed out or slept, because the next thing I remember is my mother standing in the doorway outlined by the falling sun and crying as she untied me.

Up until this point, I'd felt that she was innocent of what he'd done and that she'd just covered up for him. But as soon as I was free, I became hysterical and continued that way. Finally late that night, to quiet my crying and screaming, she, a nurse, gave me my first shot of morphine. The shots became a part of my life very quickly. I remember them threatening me, "Do you want a shot to make you behave?" The effect of morphine on a young child was almost instantly addictive. I became a junkie that day and remained hooked for the next four years. For reasons of their own, my parents would withdraw the drug at intervals and force me to quit cold turkey. I spent time in the hospital under an assumed name for a withdrawal that turned into shock and dehydration. Finally at thirteen years of age, when obtaining the drug became too hard even for them, I kicked the habit for the last time.

The next rape occurred also at thirteen. This time he caught me alone in the empty house and made a straightforward business deal: Unless I cooperated, he would rape my five-year-old sister. I submitted and, to my great shame, my body responded to him. It took me fifteen years to understand that the body will respond to stimulation no matter how revolting the source.

When I was fifteen, again in a new place, my mother left with the other children to visit her family in the East and, by design I think, left me alone in the house with him. He took no chances this time. I woke up tied to the bed. For seven days and nights he used me in any way he chose. I was allowed no time for the bathroom or anything like that. I think that by the end of the week I had become something of an animal. She apparently came home early and found me still tied. I don't know what happened to their marital life after that.

The last attack occurred when I was eighteen and pregnant with another man's child. He backed me into a corner against a counter. There was a sharp knife lying on the counter behind me. In self-defense, I stabbed him in the shoulder. The wound wasn't very deep or even serious, but it stopped him and allowed me to twist free of him. She dressed the wound for him. Then they both set out methodically to beat me. One of them (I think it was she) delivered several well-placed kicks to my stomach. The next day I miscarried my two-month-old fetus. I have had three miscarriages since then and I believe that beating had something to do with all of them. I suffered what is called a "nervous breakdown" soon after that. I attempted suicide and my psychiatrist even contemplated committing me for extended treatment. He used hypnosis and I think it helped me to submerge all of this as far as possible.

For the next several years, all of this pain and misery stayed out of conscious memory. I would wake up from a sound sleep crying but never remembered the dream that made me cry.

Finally now at age twenty-nine I have all of the pieces of myself back again. Through hypnosis and age regression, a skilled therapist gave me back my memory. If the experiences of my past taught me anything, it is that I survive.

MARTY O. DYKE

"My father thrived on the rape, battering, and emotional abuse of myself, my mother, and my sisters."

Marty O. Dyke (a pseudonym) was born in 1951 in a small town outside Albany, New York. She describes her background as "rural to suburban working class." Her poem, "Yeah I'm Blaming You," speaks of a series of violations she suffered from her father.

Marty is a lesbian separatist living in San Francisco, where she is training to be a printer.

Yeah I'm Blaming You

Yeah I'm blaming you,
You prickhole prick fuck flap jack.
I'm blaming you
And I'm blaming you *good.*
Yeah I'm telling you
You're full of shit, your "innocence"
I despise
All the drivel snivel slime grime semen-webbed
Words deeds
Creeds pleas
And pathetic lies
You've used to blazon your way through my body,
My life.

You are the rapist,
Pa.
You are the rapist whose knife I swing back burning,
You are the rot that festers this Earth.
Your poison slop filthy crap cancer trap
Pollutes this planet,
Her psyche,
Our lives.

Yeah I'm telling you
It's *all* your fault.
You done it, Dad. You
Raped me
Fucked my mother
Beat my sisters
Fucked my sisters
Raped my lovers
Beat me
And beat me.

Well listen up good now, Pa:
This daughter is raging.
                    I KNOW
                    SHE KNOWS
                    WE KNOW
                    WHAT YOU DONE
AND YEAH I'M BLAMING YOU,
You prick fuck flip fuck dick duck,
Blaming you *and* framing you
And slaying you GOOD.

PART TWO

"Yesterday I saw him watch my sister"

SURVIVORS OF SEXUAL ABUSE BY RELATIVES

LYNN SWENSON

"As I wrote this poem I began to understand my mother for the first time in my life. I now believe that she was also a victim of child sexual abuse."

Lynn Swenson (a pseudonym) was born in 1951. When she was five years old, her parents were divorced, and she and her sisters lived with their mother, who was often abusive. In all other respects she led, as she describes it, "a peculiarly sheltered and isolated life." At the age of eleven Lynn visited her grandparents' ranch. One night her grandfather molested her. Because she loved her grandmother deeply and wanted to protect her, she did not tell anyone.

The effects of this silence were far-reaching. "As a teenager I was promiscuous, somehow equating sex with affection," Lynn writes. "I also had very little self-respect. At seventeen my mother threw me out of the house. Toward the end of my seventeenth year I became pregnant and had a traumatic abortion."

Concurrent with these events, however, Lynn attempted to overcome the effects of the abuse. At fifteen she began writing poetry, finding it to be a healing experience. When she was sixteen she saw a psychiatrist and learned that simply telling someone helped her. "Gradually I became less promiscuous," she states, "and began to form relationships with men. I learned to say no. Presently I am involved with a very wonderful man."

Lynn is a recipient of grants from the National Endowment for the Arts and from the New Jersey State Council on the Arts. Her poetry has appeared in Kayak, Hanging Loose, Plum, New Jersey Monthly *and* Columbia, *and she plans to publish her first book of poetry in the near future. "From My Half-Sleep" is taken from a series of poems about her grandparents, their ranch and the desert. "At the end of the series," she writes, "there is forgiveness and an awareness of my own personal strength."*

From My Half-Sleep

From my half-sleep in the hammock
I watch my grandfather walk
to the barn, his lean legs cutting
the white expanse of sand
beyond the house. He wears levi's
and no shirt, his back sunburned
and straight, as it was.

Two years ago
I believed he was asleep,
but now I don't know.
In the still night air
he was moving chairs.
Then he came to my bed
and, reaching down, admired
my breasts under the sheet.

I remember I had never felt
blood between my legs
before that night, my grandmother
lying beside him later, innocent,
as I lay mute, the taste of his tobacco
in my mouth, my fists held tight
against my breasts, the moonlight

pouring over me,
and the thin sweat of fear.

Yesterday I saw him watch
my sister undress before the fan,
her western shirt blowing
out like sails, her thin cotton
pants caught around one foot.
Hearing his breath tighten,
I turned away. I had not told her.
I had not told anyone.

And now my grandfather
returns from the barn, a coil of rope
in his hard hand. He calls to the house
and my grandmother goes out to him.
Everywhere I look
there is blinding sand.

MAYA ANGELOU

"There was the pain. A breaking and entering when even the
senses are torn apart. The act of rape on an eight-year-old body is a
matter of the needle giving because the camel can't."

*Maya Angelou has written four autobiographical books. The ex-
cerpt reprinted here, and the epigraph above, are from the first of
these,* I Know Why the Caged Bird Sings.

Maya has also written three collections of poetry, Just Give Me
a Cool Drink of Water 'fore I Diiie, Oh Pray My Wings Are
Gonna Fit Me Well, *and* And Still I Rise. *She has worked extensively in the theater, film, and television. She produced, directed,
and starred in* Cabaret for Freedom, *starred in Genet's* The
Blacks, *adapted Sophocles'* Ajax, *and wrote and produced a ten-
part TV series on African traditions in American life.*

*At the request of Dr. Martin Luther King, Jr., she became the
northern coordinator for the Southern Christian Leadership Conference. In 1975 she received the* Ladies' Home Journal *Woman
of the Year Award in communications. President Carter appoint-
ed her to the Commission of International Women's Year and
she is on the board of trustees of the American Film Institute. She
is one of the few women members of the Directors Guild and is
the author of the television screenplays* The Sisters *and* I Know
Why the Caged Bird Sings.

120

from I Know Why the Caged Bird Sings

I had decided that St. Louis was a foreign country. I would never get used to the scurrying sounds of flushing toilets, or the packaged foods, or doorbells or the noise of cars and trains and buses that crashed through the walls or slipped under the doors. In my mind I only stayed in St. Louis for a few weeks. As quickly as I understood that I had not reached my home, I sneaked away to Robin Hood's forest and the caves of Alley Oop where all reality was unreal and even that changed every day. I carried the same shield that I had used in Stamps: "I didn't come to stay."

Mother was competent in providing for us. Even if that meant getting someone else to furnish the provisions. Although she was a nurse, she never worked at her profession while we were with her. Mr. Freeman brought in the necessities and she earned extra money cutting poker games in the gambling parlors. The straight eight-to-five world simply didn't have enough glamour for her, and it was twenty years later that I first saw her in a nurse's uniform.

Mr. Freeman was a foreman in the Southern Pacific yards and came home late sometimes, after Mother had gone out. He took his dinner off the stove where she had carefully covered it and which she had admonished us not to bother. He ate quietly in the kitchen while Bailey and I read separately and greedily our own Street and Smith pulp magazine. Now that we had spending money, we bought the illustrated paperbacks with their gaudy pictures. When Mother was away, we were put on an honor system. We had to finish our homework, eat dinner and wash the dishes before we could read or listen to *The Lone Ranger, Crime Busters* or *The Shadow*.

Mr. Freeman moved gracefully, like a big brown bear, and seldom spoke to us. He simply waited for Mother and put his whole self into the waiting. He never read the paper or patted his foot to radio. He waited. That was all.

If she came home before we went to bed, we saw the man come alive. He would start out of the big chair, like a man coming out of sleep, smiling. I would remember then that a few seconds before, I had heard a car door slam; then Mother's footsteps would signal from the concrete walk. When her key rattled the door, Mr. Freeman would have already asked his habitual question, "Hey, Bibbi, have a good time?"

His query would hang in the air while she sprang over to peck him on the lips. Then she turned to Bailey and me with the lipstick kisses. "Haven't you finished your homework?" If we had and were just reading—"O.K., say your prayers and go to bed." If we hadn't—"Then go to your room and finish . . . then say your prayers and go to bed."

Mr. Freeman's smile never grew, it stayed at the same intensity. Sometimes Mother would go over and sit on his lap and the grin on his face looked as if it would stay there forever.

From our rooms we could hear the glasses clink and the radio turned up. I think she must have danced for him on the good nights, because he couldn't dance, but before I fell asleep I often heard feet shuffling to dance rhythms.

I felt very sorry for Mr. Freeman. I felt as sorry for him as I had felt for a litter of helpless pigs born in our backyard sty in Arkansas. We fattened the pigs all year long for the slaughter on the first good frost, and even as I suffered for the cute little wiggly things, I knew how much I was going to enjoy the fresh sausage and hog's headcheese they could give me only with their deaths.

Because of the lurid tales we read and our vivid imaginations and, probably, memories of our brief but hectic lives, Bailey and I were afflicted—he physically and I mentally. He stuttered, and I sweated through horrifying nightmares. He was constantly told to slow down and start again, and on my particularly bad nights my mother would take me in to sleep with her, in the large bed with Mr. Freeman.

Because of a need for stability, children easily become creatures of habit. After the third time in Mother's bed, I thought there was nothing strange about sleeping there.

One morning she got out of bed for an early errand, and I fell asleep again. But I awoke to a pressure, a strange feeling on my left leg. It was too soft to be a hand, and it wasn't the touch of clothes. Whatever it was, I hadn't encountered the sensation in all the years of sleeping with Momma. It didn't move, and I was too startled to. I turned my head a little to the left to see if Mr. Freeman was awake and gone, but his eyes were open and both hands were above the cover. I knew, as I had always known, it was his "thing" on my leg.

He said, "Just stay right here, Ritie, I ain't gonna hurt you." I wasn't afraid, a little apprehensive, maybe, but not afraid. Of course I knew that lots of people did "it" and they used their "things" to accomplish the deed, but no one I knew had ever done it to anybody. Mr. Freeman pulled me to him and put his hand between my legs. He didn't hurt, but Momma had drilled into my head: "Keep your legs closed, and don't let nobody see your pocketbook."

"Now, I didn't hurt you. Don't get scared." He threw back the blankets and his "thing" stood up like a brown ear of corn. He took my hand and said, "Feel it." It was mushy and squirmy like the inside of a freshly killed chicken. Then he dragged me on top of his chest with his left arm, and his right hand was moving so fast and his heart was beating so hard that I was afraid that he would die. Ghost stories revealed how people who died wouldn't let go of whatever they were holding. I wondered if Mr. Freeman died holding me how I would ever get free. Would they have to break his arms to get me loose?

Finally he was quiet, and then came the nice part. He held me so softly that I wished he wouldn't ever let me go. I felt at home. From the way he was holding me I knew he'd never let me go or let anything bad ever happen to me. This was probably my real father and we had found each other at last. But then he rolled over, leaving me in a wet place, and stood up.

"I gotta talk to you, Ritie." He pulled off his shorts that had fallen to his ankles, and went into the bathroom.

It was true the bed was wet, but I knew I hadn't had an accident. Maybe Mr. Freeman had one while he was holding me. He came back with a glass of water and told me in a sour voice, "Get up. You peed in the bed." He poured water on the wet spot and it did look like my mattress on many mornings.

Having lived in Southern strictness, I knew when to keep quiet around adults, but I did want to ask him why he said I peed when I was sure he didn't believe that. If he thought I was naughty, would that mean that he would never hold me again? Or admit that he was my father? I had made him ashamed of me.

"Ritie, you love Bailey." He sat down on the bed and I came close, hoping. "Yes." He was bending down, pulling on his socks, and his back was so large and friendly I wanted to rest my head on it.

"If you ever tell anybody what we did, I'll have to kill Bailey."

What had we done? We? Obviously he didn't mean my peeing in the bed. I didn't understand and didn't dare ask him. It had something to do with his holding me. But there was no chance to ask Bailey either, because that would be telling what we had done. The thought that he might kill Bailey stunned me. After he left the room I thought about telling Mother that I hadn't peed in the bed, but then if she asked me what happened I'd have to tell her about Mr. Freeman holding me, and that wouldn't do.

It was the same old quandary. I had always lived it. There was an army of adults, whose motives and movements I just couldn't understand and who made no effort to understand mine. There was never any question of my disliking Mr. Freeman, I simply didn't understand him either.

For weeks after, he said nothing to me, except the gruff hellos which were given without ever looking in my direction.

This was the first secret I had ever kept from Bailey and sometimes I thought he should be able to read it on my face, but he noticed nothing.

I began to feel lonely for Mr. Freeman and the encasement of his big arms. Before, my world had been Bailey, food, Momma, the Store, reading books and Uncle Willie. Now, for the first time, it included physical contact.

I began to wait for Mr. Freeman to come in from the yards, but when he did, he never noticed me, although I put a lot of feeling into "Good evening, Mr. Freeman."

One evening, when I couldn't concentrate on anything, I went over to him and sat quickly on his lap. He had been waiting for Mother again. Bailey was listening to *The Shadow* and didn't miss me. At first Mr. Freeman sat still, not holding me or anything, then I felt a soft lump under my thigh begin to move. It twitched against me and started to harden. Then he pulled me to his chest. He smelled of coal dust and grease and he was so close I buried my face in his shirt and listened to his heart, it was beating just for me. Only I could hear the thud, only I could feel the jumping on my face. He said, "Sit still, stop squirming." But all the time, he pushed me around on his lap, then suddenly he stood up and I slipped down to the floor. He ran to the bathroom.

For months he stopped speaking to me again. I was hurt and for a time felt lonelier than ever. But then I forgot about him, and even the memory of his holding me precious melted into the general darkness just beyond the great blinkers of childhood.

I read more than ever, and wished my soul that I had been born a boy. Horatio Alger was the greatest writer in the world. His heroes were always good, always won, and were always boys. I could have developed the first two virtues, but becoming a boy was sure to be difficult, if not impossible.

The Sunday funnies influenced me, and although I admired the strong heroes who always conquered in the end, I identified with Tiny Tim. In the toilet, where I used to take the papers, it was tortuous to look for and exclude the unnecessary pages so that I could learn how he would finally outwit his latest adversary. I wept with relief every Sunday as he eluded the evil men and bounded back from each seeming defeat as sweet and gentle as ever. The Katzenjammer kids were fun because they made the adults look stupid. But they were a little too smart-alecky for my taste.

When spring came to St. Louis, I took out my first library card, and since Bailey and I seemed to be growing apart, I spent most of my Saturdays at the library (no interruptions) breathing in the world of penniless shoeshine boys who, with goodness and perseverance, became rich, rich men, and gave baskets of goodies to the poor on holidays. The little princesses who were mistaken for maids, and the long-lost children mistaken for waifs, became more real to me than our house, our mother, our school or Mr. Freeman.

During those months we saw our grandparents and the uncles (our only aunt had gone to California to build her fortune), but they usually asked the same question, "Have you been good children?" for which there was only one answer. Even Bailey wouldn't have dared to answer no.

On a late spring Saturday, after our chores (nothing like those in Stamps) were done, Bailey and I were going out, he to play baseball and I to the library. Mr. Freeman said to me, after Bailey had gone downstairs, "Ritie, go get some milk for the house."

Mother usually brought milk when she came in, but that morning as Bailey and I straightened the living room her bedroom door had been open, and we knew that she hadn't come home the night before.

He gave me the money and I rushed to the store and back to the house. After putting the milk in the icebox, I turned and had just reached the front door when I heard "Ritie." He was sitting in the big chair by the radio. "Ritie, come here." I didn't think about the holding time until I got close to him. His pants were open and his "thing" was standing out of his britches by itself.

"No, sir, Mr. Freeman." I started to back away. I didn't want to touch that mushy-hard thing again, and I didn't need him to hold me anymore. He grabbed my arm and pulled me between his legs. His face was still and looked kind, but he didn't smile or blink his eyes. Nothing. He did nothing, except reach his left hand around to turn on the radio without even looking at it. Over the noise of music and static, he said, "Now, this ain't gonna hurt you much. You liked it before, didn't you?"

I didn't want to admit that I had in fact liked his holding me or that I had liked his smell or the hard heartbeating, so I said nothing. And his face became like the face of those mean natives the Phantom was always having to beat up.

His legs were squeezing my waist. "Pull down your drawers." I hesitated for two reasons: he was holding me too tight to move, and I was sure that any minute my mother or Bailey or the Green Hornet would bust in the door and save me.

"We was just playing before." He released me enough to snatch down my bloomers, and then he dragged me closer to him. Turning the radio up loud, too loud, he said, "If you scream, I'm gonna kill you. And if you tell, I'm gonna kill Bailey." I could tell he meant what he said. I couldn't understand why he wanted to kill my brother. Neither of us had done anything to him. And then.

Then there was the pain. A breaking and entering when even the senses are torn apart. The act of rape on an eight-year-old body is a matter of the needle giving because the camel can't. The child gives, because the body can, and the mind of the violator cannot.

I thought I had died—I woke up in a white-walled world, and it had to be heaven. But Mr. Freeman was there and he was washing me. His hands shook, but he held me upright in the tub and washed my legs. "I didn't mean to hurt you, Ritie. I didn't mean it. But don't you tell. . . . Remember, don't you tell a soul."

I felt cool and very clean and just a little tired. "No, sir, Mr. Freeman, I won't tell." I was somewhere above everything. "It's just that I'm so tired I'll just go and lay down a while, please," I whispered to him. I thought if I spoke out loud, he might become frightened and hurt me again. He dried me and handed me my bloomers. "Put these on and go to the library. Your momma ought to be coming home soon. You just act natural."

Walking down the street, I felt the wet on my pants, and my hips seemed to be coming out of their sockets. I couldn't sit long on the hard seats in the library (they had been constructed for children), so I walked by the empty lot where Bailey was playing ball, but he wasn't there. I stood for a while and watched the big boys tear around the dusty diamond and then headed for home.

After two blocks, I knew I'd never make it. Not unless I counted every step and stepped on every crack. I had started to burn between my legs more than the time I'd wasted Sloan's Liniment on myself. My legs throbbed, or rather the insides of my thighs throbbed, with the same force that Mr. Freeman's heart had beaten. Thrum . . . step . . . thrum . . . step . . . STEP ON THE CRACK . . . thrum . . . step. I went up the stairs one at a time. No one was in the living room, so I went straight to bed, after hiding my red-and-yellow-stained drawers under the mattress.

When Mother came in she said, "Well, young lady, I believe this is the first time I've seen you go to bed without being told. You must be sick."

I wasn't sick, but the pit of my stomach was on fire—how could I tell her that? Bailey came in later and asked me what the matter was. There was nothing to tell him. When Mother called us to eat and I said I wasn't hungry, she laid her cool hand on my forehead and cheeks. "Maybe it's the measles. They say they're going around the neighborhood." After she took my temperature she said, "You have a little fever. You've probably just caught them."

Mr. Freeman took up the whole doorway. "Then Bailey ought not to be in there with her. Unless you want a house full of sick children." She answered over her shoulder, "He may as well have them now as later. Get them over with." She brushed by Mr. Freeman as if he were made of cotton. "Come on, Junior. Get some cool towels and wipe your sister's face."

As Bailey left the room, Mr. Freeman advanced to the bed. He leaned over, his whole face a threat that could have smothered me. "If you tell . . ." And again so softly, I almost didn't hear it— "If you tell." I couldn't summon up the energy to answer him. He had to know that I wasn't going to tell anything. Bailey came in with the towels and Mr. Freeman walked out.

Later Mother made a broth and sat on the edge of the bed to feed me. The liquid went down my throat like bones. My belly and behind were as heavy as cold iron, but it seemed my head had gone away and pure air had replaced it on my shoulders. Bailey read to me from *The Rover Boys* until he got sleepy and went to bed.

That night I kept waking to hear Mother and Mr. Freeman arguing. I couldn't hear what they were saying, but I did hope that she wouldn't make him so mad that he'd hurt her too. I knew he could do it, with his cold face and empty eyes. Their voices came in faster and faster, the high sounds on the heels of the lows. I would have liked to have gone in. Just passed through as if I were going to the toilet. Just show my face and they might stop, but my legs refused to move. I could move the toes and ankles, but the knees had turned to wood.

Maybe I slept, but soon morning was there and Mother was pretty over my bed. "How're you feeling, baby?"

"Fine, Mother." An instinctive answer. "Where's Bailey?"

She said he was still asleep but that she hadn't slept all night. She had been in my room off and on to see about me. I asked her where Mr. Freeman was, and her face chilled with remembered anger. "He's gone. Moved this morning. I'm going to take your temperature after I put on your Cream of Wheat."

Could I tell her now? The terrible pain assured me that I couldn't. What he did to me, and what I allowed, must have been very bad if already God let me hurt so much. If Mr. Freeman was gone, did that mean Bailey was out of danger? And if so, if I told him, would he still love me?

After Mother took my temperature, she said she was going to bed for a while but to wake her if I felt sicker. She told Bailey to watch my face and arms for spots and when they came up he could paint them with calamine lotion.

That Sunday goes and comes in my memory like a bad connection on an overseas telephone call. Once, Bailey was reading *The Katzenjammer Kids* to me, and then without a pause for sleeping, Mother was looking closely at my face and soup trickled down my chin and some got into my mouth and I choked. Then there was a doctor who took my temperature and held my wrist.

"Bailey!" I supposed I had screamed, for he materialized suddenly, and I asked him to help me and we'd run away to California or France or Chicago. I knew that I was dying and, in fact, I longed for death, but I didn't want to die anywhere near Mr. Freeman. I knew that even now he wouldn't have allowed death to have me unless he wished it to.

Mother said I should be bathed and the linens had to be changed since I had sweat so much. But when they tried to move me I fought, and even Bailey couldn't hold me. Then she picked me up in her arms and the terror abated for a while. Bailey began to change the bed. As he pulled off the soiled sheets, he dislodged the panties I had put under the mattress. They fell at Mother's feet.

In the hospital, Bailey told me that I had to tell who did that to me, or the man would hurt another little girl. When I explained that I couldn't tell because the man would kill him, Bailey said knowingly, "He can't kill me. I won't let him." And of course I believed him. Bailey didn't lie to me. So I told him.

Bailey cried at the side of my bed until I started to cry too. Almost fifteen years passed before I saw my brother cry again.

Using the old brain he was born with (those were his words later on that day), he gave his information to Grandmother Baxter, and Mr. Freeman was arrested and was spared the awful wrath of my pistol-whipping uncles.

I would have liked to stay in the hospital the rest of my life. Mother brought flowers and candy. Grandmother came with fruit and my uncles clumped around and around my bed, snorting like wild horses. When they were able to sneak Bailey in, he read to me for hours.

The saying that people who have nothing to do become busybodies is not the only truth. Excitement is a drug, and people whose lives are filled with violence are always wondering where the next "fix" is coming from.

The court was filled. Some people even stood behind the churchlike benches in the rear. Overhead fans moved with the detachment of old men. Grandmother Baxter's clients were there in gay and flippant array. The gamblers in pin-striped suits and their makeup-deep women whispered to me out of blood-red mouths that now I knew as much as they did. I was eight, and grown. Even the nurses in the hospital had told me that now I had nothing to fear. "The worst is over for you," they had said. So I put the words in all the smirking mouths.

I sat with my family (Bailey couldn't come) and they rested still on the seats like solid, cold gray tombstones. Thick and forevermore unmoving.

"What was the defendant wearing?" That was Mr. Freeman's lawyer.

"I don't know."

"You mean to say this man raped you and you don't know what he was wearing?" He snickered as if I had raped Mr. Freeman. "Do you know if you were raped?"

A sound pushed in the air of the court (I was sure it was laughter). I was glad that Mother had let me wear the navy blue winter coat with brass buttons. Although it was too short and the weather was typical St. Louis hot, the coat was a friend that I hugged to me in the strange and unfriendly place.

"Was that the first time the accused touched you?" The question stopped me. Mr. Freeman had surely done something very wrong, but I was convinced that I had helped him to do it. I didn't want to lie, but the lawyer wouldn't let me think, so I used silence as a retreat.

"Did the accused try to touch you before the time he or rather you say he raped you?"

I couldn't say yes and tell them how he had loved me once for a few minutes and how he had held me close before he thought I had peed in my bed. My uncles would kill me and Grandmother Baxter would stop speaking, as she often did when she was angry. And all those people in the court would stone me as they had stoned the harlot in the Bible. And Mother, who thought I was such a good girl, would be so disappointed. But most important, there was Bailey. I had kept a big secret from him.

"Marguerite, answer the question. Did the accused touch you before the occasion on which you claim he raped you?"

Everyone in the court knew that the answer had to be No. Everyone except Mr. Freeman and me. I looked at his heavy face trying to look as if he would have liked me to say No. I said No.

The lie lumped in my throat and I couldn't get air. How I despised the man for making me lie. Old, mean, nasty thing. Old, black, nasty thing. The tears didn't soothe my heart as they usually did. I screamed, "Ole, mean, dirty thing, you. Dirty old thing." Our lawyer brought me off the stand and to my mother's arms. The fact that I had arrived at my desired destination by lies made it less appealing to me.

Mr. Freeman was given one year and one day, but he never got a chance to do his time. His lawyer (or someone) got him released that very afternoon.

In the living room, where the shades were drawn for coolness, Bailey and I played Monopoly on the floor. I played a bad game because I was thinking how I would be able to tell Bailey how I had lied and, even worse for our relationship, kept a secret from him. Bailey answered the doorbell, because Grandmother was in the kitchen. A tall white policeman asked for Mrs. Baxter. Had they found out about the lie? Maybe the policeman was coming to put me in jail because I had sworn on the Bible that everything I said would be the truth, the whole truth, so help me, God. The man in our living room was taller than the sky and whiter than my image of God. He just didn't have the beard.

"Mrs. Baxter, I thought you ought to know. Freeman's been found dead on the lot behind the slaughterhouse." Softly, as if she were discussing a church program, she said, "Poor man." She wiped her hands on the dish towel and just as softly asked, "Do they know who did it?"

The policeman said, "Seems like he was dropped there. Some say he was kicked to death."

Grandmother's color only rose a little. "Tom, thanks for telling me. Poor man. Well, maybe it's better this way. He *was* a mad dog. Would you like a glass of lemonade? Or some beer?"

Although he looked harmless, I knew he was a dreadful angel counting out my many sins.

"No, thanks, Mrs. Baxter. I'm on duty. Gotta be getting back."

"Well, tell your ma that I'll be over when I take up my beer and remind her to save some kraut for me."

And the recording angel was gone. He was gone, and a man was dead because I lied. Where was the balance in that? One lie surely wouldn't be worth a man's life. Bailey could have explained it all to me, but I didn't dare ask him. Obviously I had forfeited my place in heaven forever, and I was as gutless as the doll I had ripped to pieces ages ago. Even Christ Himself turned His back on Satan. Wouldn't He turn His back on me? I could feel the evilness flowing through my body and waiting, pent up, to rush off my tongue if I tried to open my mouth. I clamped my teeth shut, I'd hold it in. If it escaped, wouldn't it flood the world and all the innocent people?

Grandmother Baxter said, "Ritie and Junior, you didn't hear a thing. I never want to hear this situation or that evil man's name mentioned in my house again. I mean that." She went back into the kitchen to make apple strudel for my celebration.

Even Bailey was frightened. He sat all to himself, looking at a man's death—a kitten looking at a wolf. Not quite understanding it but frightened all the same.

In those moments I decided that although Bailey loved me, he couldn't help. I had sold myself to the Devil and there could be no escape. The only thing I could do was to stop talking to people other than Bailey. Instinctively, or somehow, I knew that because I loved him so much I'd never hurt him, but if I talked to anyone else, that person might die too. Just my breath, carrying my words out, might poison people and they'd curl up and die like the black fat slugs that only pretended.

I had to stop talking.

I discovered that to achieve perfect personal silence all I had to do was to attach myself leechlike to sound. I began to listen to everything. I probably hoped that after I had heard all the sounds, really heard them and packed them down, deep in my ears, the world would be quiet around me. I walked into rooms where people were laughing, their voices hitting the walls like stones, and I simply stood still—in the midst of the riot of sound. After a minute or two, silence would rush into the room from its hiding place because I had eaten up all the sounds.

In the first weeks my family accepted my behavior as a post-rape, post-hospital affliction. (Neither the term nor the experience was mentioned in Grandmother's house, where Bailey and I were again staying.) They understood that I could talk to Bailey, but to no one else.

Then came the last visit from the visiting nurse, and the doctor said I was healed. That meant that I should be back on the sidewalks playing handball or enjoying the games I had been given when I was sick. When I refused to be the child they knew and accepted me to be, I was called impudent and my muteness sullenness.

For a while I was punished for being so uppity that I wouldn't speak; and then came the thrashings, given by any relative who felt himself offended.

We were on the train going back to Stamps, and this time it was I who had to console Bailey. He cried his heart out down the aisles of the coach, and pressed his little-boy body against the windowpane looking for a last glimpse of his Mother Dear.

I have never known if Momma sent for us, or if the St. Louis family just got fed up with my grim presence. There is nothing more appalling than a constantly morose child.

I cared less about the trip than about the fact that Bailey was unhappy, and had no more thought of our destination than if I had simply been heading for the toilet.

The barrenness of Stamps was exactly what I wanted, without will or consciousness. After St. Louis, with its noise and activity, its trucks and buses, and loud family gatherings, I welcomed the obscure lanes and lonely bungalows set back deep in dirt yards.

The resignation of its inhabitants encouraged me to relax. They showed me a contentment based on the belief that nothing more was coming to them, although a great deal more was due. Their decision to be satisfied with life's inequities was a lesson for me. Entering Stamps, I had the feeling that I was stepping over the border lines of the map and would fall, without fear, right off the end of the world. Nothing more could happen, for in Stamps nothing happened.

Into this cocoon I crept.

BLANCHE WOODBURY

"I now believe and *feel* that I am a true survivor, not a victim of my brother and my guilt."

Blanche Woodbury (a pseudonym) was born in 1952 in a small, rural town in Connecticut. When Blanche was an infant her mother suffered a nervous breakdown and committed herself to a psychiatric care center. Blanche's grandmother came to take care of Blanche and her older brother. In looking back, it seems to Blanche that their mother's absence must have been particularly difficult for her brother: "To me it was normal to have a weekend mother, but he had been used to always having her at home. Several times my mother has related to me the account a neighbor gave to her of a conversation this woman had with my brother. He was six or seven at the time, I was a year old and he was wheeling me about the lawn in my baby carriage. 'You must love your little sister very much,' the neighbor said to him. 'No,' he said. 'Why do you say that?' the neighbor asked. 'Because of what she did to my mother!' my brother said.

When Blanche was six and he was twelve, her brother began sexually abusing her and continued to do so for five years. It stopped when their grandmother found them naked one afternoon in her brother's bedroom. Her grandmother began to beat Blanche. "How long? It seemed forever," Blanche writes. "I have blotted out of my memory what happened next."

As an adult she suppressed memories of the abuse and poured her energies into becoming an achiever: "A's in school, publication of my writing... always the search for redemption." Then

136

*one night for no apparent reason Blanche drank to such an extent
that she was hospitalized for two days. She began seeing a psychologist for help in dealing with the incest. Her goal is to be able
to talk to her brother about her pain. "Perhaps I will be able to
give him a copy of this anthology as my first overture of communication," she concludes.*

My Brother

My brother lives in a box of cigars.
Each day every day
he lifts the lid to peek at the world
and hopes the world won't notice.
Bristles grow on his face and throat.
He smells, fears soap.
He never throws his loose hairs away
but carefully keeps them, dirty and dark,
in the teeth of a green plastic comb.

Long ago he spent years committing incest.
I survived but we never mention it.
He's thirty-five now and still lives with our mother.
My favorite joke when I visit is to talk
of the time I stabbed his thigh with a fork
and sent him screeching around the table
for ruining my first perfect crayoned picture.
We pretend to laugh and the scar
does not go away. Migraine headaches
take me back to the fork, to the fort
he built under cool pines

where he wouldn't let me visit
unless I would and I did.

Now he does his best to repel.
He rots his teeth, sucks his cigars,
growls and belches and gets fat.
Each night every night
he grows a little smaller inside.
One morning my mother, weeping,
may find he's flickered out at last,
a tiny gray heap in an ashtray.
I'll visit, leave the jokes behind,
bring instead a perfect crayoned picture
to wrap around his coffin.

DESI

"I came to think of a woman's touch as meaning pain and fear and all the old feelings I knew so well as a child."

Desi was born in the early Fifties in a small town in Pennsylvania. As a young child, she was sexually abused by her grandmother. Throughout childhood and adolescence, she distrusted women. "I was very open about how I hated women," she says. She preferred instead to be with men.

When she was nineteen, Desi met a woman who is still her best friend, and this friendship enabled her to begin to trust women again. "I realize now that my grandmother was very sick," she states. "It had nothing to do with my being 'a bad girl' when I was little, as I used to think."

During her weekly visits, Desi's grandmother has continued to disapprove of Desi and her refusal to be like the other females in the family, who are all male-identified. "It has made her furious that I don't worship men, that I do not depend on them for approval or ego gratification, and that I love women and have built my life on being a radical feminist woman who loves her sisters."

She concludes, "My grandmother has been brainwashed by the patriarchy, and it was very sad and horrible that she inflicted it on me."

Story of a Granddaughter

From the time I was five until I was seven, my grandmother took care of me weekends when my parents went out. She gave me my bath and put me to bed. I dreaded this. She had the idea that female genitals smelled and you had to be constantly washing yourself. She was always telling me how women "smell bad," how even if you wash it's always there.

I should say here that my grandmother hated women and absolutely worshiped men and everything they did. To her, a man couldn't do any wrong. She didn't even blame men for rape and women-battering; she said that the women "asked for it."

When she gave me my bath, she made me lie back in the tub and spread my legs while she separated my genitals with her fingers. She used a washcloth first, then she dropped that and used her hand, which was extremely painful because she had long fingernails. When I cried, she told me to be quiet, that if she didn't get me clean I'd smell. She threatened to spank me or tell my parents what a bad girl I'd been.

As I was easily intimidated, I tried to stop crying and hoped that the bath would be over soon. But she continued on and was even rougher with me as punishment. I couldn't understand why she was doing this. When I washed myself, it didn't hurt; it only hurt when she washed me. I thought maybe she knew I masturbated in bed at night and was punishing me for that. After the bath, she took a towel and dried me very roughly, and sometimes she splashed some kind of after-bath cologne on me, which stung like hell.

One time after she did that, I got out of bed to go to the bathroom to urinate and found that I couldn't, there was a terrible searing pain. I was scared and yet I couldn't tell my parents, because I knew they'd think I was lying. I knew they'd believe my grandmother because I was just a child. I kept wondering what she was punishing me for and why she didn't love me, although at other times she was very loving and generous with gifts. I remember that night being scared that I'd never be able to "go pee" again and wondering if I was going to die. I was okay by the next day except for a little soreness, so no permanent damage was done. No physical damage, anyway.

I don't recall her ever making penetration (although sometimes it felt like she was trying to get inside me to wipe out all traces of odor) and I never bled after she was done. I'd just feel scraped, ripped, and frightened. I tried to get her to stop by telling her I loved her and by putting my arms around her neck, but that didn't work. She told me she loved me too, and that I had to be a clean little girl or people wouldn't want to be near me. I kept wondering why my mother never did that to me when she bathed me, or why my father never did on the occasions when he was in charge of my bath.

There was one time when she used a Q-Tip cotton swab on me after my bath and it felt like she was trying to get inside me with that. All I remember was how she kept poking with it and how it hurt so bad. I had moments of feeling it was my own fault, and I went through a short period of being real good all the time (totally mystifying my parents) as though trying to make sure nothing like that would happen to me again.

LOUISE THORNTON

"Sometimes I still imagine Uncle Karl sitting by the kitchen table."

Louise Thornton, who was born in 1941, wrote "Uncle Karl" out of an attempt to understand child sexual abuse within her family. While it did not involve her directly, it caused her grief: "I wanted to show that the effects of this abuse are far-reaching. They extend beyond the child and the person who abused her or him. Child sexual abuse is a betrayal of anyone who trusts others. And how can we live without trust?

"I wish I had been able to speak to Uncle Karl about what he did," she continues. "This could have enabled each of us to be with each other who we really are, to forgive, to be healed. I continue the process without him but with the help of friends. The healing is often slow and uneven. But I feel much closer to reaching a peace both with Uncle Karl and with myself, and I am grateful."

In 1989 *Louise Thornton co-edited* Touching Fire: Erotic Writings By Women, *published by Carroll and Graf.*

Uncle Karl

Early one summer morning when I was four, a man I did not know opened the kitchen screen door. He was wearing a soldier's dark uniform and a soldier's hat. The train whistle faded down the railroad tracks, and still he stood there, hesitant. Then he took a step forward, and his shadow fell across the doorsill, reaching out into the room. I dashed under the table to hide.

My mother ran into the kitchen from the pantry. "It's your uncle Karl!" she cried. "He's come home from the war."

The man went to my mother and hugged her. "I just got off the train from Chicago," he said. "I came here first. I couldn't wait to see you and Lollie!"

After that, Uncle Karl was almost as much a part of the family as my mother and father and my young brother, Frank. Once or twice a week he would stop by for a cup of coffee, sitting by the white kitchen table, chair tilted, cap pushed back on his head, a cigarette balanced between two fingers.

Uncle Karl's bachelor house was set back from the gravel road in a field of clover. Often he invited the family to come and listen to his old dance-band records. At these times my mother, Aunt Lydia, and Uncle Karl laughed and talked about how it was when they were all small and home together. After Uncle Karl told a new story about his mischievousness as a boy, my father slapped him on the back, shouting, "You old son of a gun!" Our cousin Jeffrey, Frank, and I sat quietly and smiled at each other, knowing that eventually Uncle Karl would remember to get out the chocolate cookies with vanilla frosting. When the records were played, I took Jeffrey by the hand and we galloped around the living room in time to the music while Frank giggled in the doorway. Our world was infinitely beautiful then.

The year I was eight, Uncle Karl organized a family picnic on the Fourth of July, setting up a huge tent in a grassy field and inviting everyone, including third and fourth cousins. My cousin Claire and her family came all the way from Oregon. I was overjoyed. While Claire lived so distant that we saw each other only once a year, she was my best friend. I had other friends in school, but I did not feel that I could tell them everything. They would not begin to understand my shy, quiet mother or my angry father. But Claire did. Her family was almost like mine.

At the picnic, music played from the speakers Uncle Karl had set up inside and outside the tent while firecrackers banged in staccato thunderings all around us. Claire, my other girl cousins, and I streamed in and out of the tent, a piece of chicken in one hand and a soda in the other. Uncle Karl teased Frank or Jeffrey, running his hand across their heads and smiling broadly. Once when I glanced into a dark corner of the tent, Uncle Karl was pulling Jeffrey onto his lap. He was seven then and I think felt too old for such things. Jeffrey fell into it, his face turning a deep red. Later, Claire and I came across Jeffrey sitting in Aunt Lydia and Uncle Joe's car by himself. He looked as if he had been crying.

"What do you think is the matter with him?" I asked Claire.

"Oh, nothing! He acts like such a baby sometimes!"

I shrugged my shoulders. "I guess you're right."

Finally it was night and time for Uncle Karl to set off the fireworks he had been accumulating for months. Wheels of fire whirled round and round; rockets shot up into the black sky with a whoosh; pink and orange blossoms exploded high above us, drifting back down to earth in separate petals. For the finale, Uncle Karl ignited a series of missiles and cannons that roared and shrieked against the night for three or four minutes. Then, suddenly, it was over. Millions of miles above us, the silent stars reclaimed the silent sky.

"That was an incredible show!" my father exclaimed to Uncle Karl as we climbed into the car to go home.

"It was, wasn't it?" he answered. "But wait until next year. It will be even better."

Then one Sunday afternoon when I was nine and Frank eight, Uncle Karl stopped at our house on his way home from church. It seemed strange, as he had just been there the night before. "I'm going to the stock-car races in Timby," he said. "I thought Frank might like to come along. Would you, Frank?"

"Sure!" Frank answered. "I've always wanted to see a race."

Uncle Karl put his arm around Frank's shoulders. "I thought so. We'll have a good time."

"Couldn't I go, too?" I begged. "Please, Uncle Karl?"

"This is just for boys. You wouldn't like all that dirt and noise anyway. C'mon, Frank. We have a date!" They drove away together.

After the two of them had gone to the races for the third time, I complained. "Just because I'm a girl, I have to stay home," I said to my mother. "It isn't fair! And what is there to do around here? Nothing!"

My mother looked directly into my eyes. "Be glad for Frank," she said. "Your father doesn't know how to be friends with him. He's either mad at Frank for something he did or too busy to even notice him. At least Uncle Karl enjoys being with Frank."

Soon Uncle Karl was taking Frank everywhere. In the winter they tramped through the fields hunting. On warm spring evenings they watched drive-in movies. In summer they strolled through carnivals stretching down the entire length of Main Street, the Ferris wheel spinning through the dark nights like a hundred twinkling stars. I watched these lights from my front porch, completely miserable.

As I grew older and became preoccupied with school activities, I no longer missed this special attention. Uncle Karl continued to visit often, but Frank did not go away with him as much as before. Once they planned to take a trip to Colorado together, leaving immediately after school was out on Friday, but Frank did not come home. When it grew dark, Uncle Karl left without him. At midnight Frank crept in the door and asked anxiously, "Is Uncle Karl gone?"

"He couldn't wait forever!" our father roared. "You had no business staying out so late." He gave him a kick. "Go to bed!"

Frank looked relieved and ran up the stairs. I could not understand it. How could Frank not want to go with Uncle Karl?

Another time Uncle Karl invited Frank to a movie, but Frank had acquired a job in the grocery store and said that he was too tired after work to go anywhere.

"I'll go!" I said quickly. "Couldn't I?"

"Well," Uncle Karl answered, "I told your cousin Jeffrey he could come with me if Frank didn't want to. I hate to turn him down after I already invited him. You know how Aunt Lydia is. She won't let that boy do anything! And Joe does nothing but sit in a chair and sleep. Jeffrey used to be a crybaby, but he's growing up. He can't wait to go along with me."

I did not ask again.

Then it was the summer of my thirteenth year. One day I came home to find Uncle Karl waiting for me by the kitchen table. "I'm driving to Oregon to visit James and Irene. Would you like to come along and see Claire?"

I could not believe it. After all these years, he was asking me. I looked at my mother. "It's a wonderful chance to see your cousin," she said. "Why don't you go?"

We drove into the night. Crickets throbbed in the still, moist air. I said very little, but Uncle Karl did not seem to mind. Around other adults I always felt uncomfortable, as if they were waiting for me to say something. With Uncle Karl I felt relaxed. He drove carefully, listening to the quiet hum of the car radio playing country-western songs. After a long while he said, "You know what I've always wanted to do?"

"No. What?"

"Get in the car some evening just like we are now, start driving down any road, and never stop."

"Never?"

He laughed. "Never. Just go where the car took you. Wouldn't that be fun?"

The road stretched ahead of us, the cool, white line down the center reaching into the darkness. I imagined it going on forever. "It would!" I answered. "I can't think of anything that would be more fun."

"Shall we do it sometime?"

"I'd love to!" I knew we were kidding each other. But I also knew that each of us, in a secret part of our heart, meant it entirely.

Claire and I had a wonderful visit. We were best friends again, sharing everything. On Sunday afternoon Uncle Karl and I drove home. All the way back I thought that no one could possibly have a better uncle than Uncle Karl.

Almost before I knew it, I was eighteen and my last year at home was coming to an end. After graduation I would be leaving for college in a distant state. While I was anxious to leave the constricting smallness of my hometown, I was also afraid. Who did I think I was, wanting a college education when no one in my family had ever obtained more than a high-school diploma? Even Claire had married and settled a few miles from her parents. I would be leaving everyone behind. And while my father had encouraged me to enroll in college, my mother already mourned my departure.

Graduation night came, we marched solemnly down the aisle to "Pomp and Circumstance," and it was over. I found myself alone outside the auditorium, my mother and father having hurried home to prepare cake and ice cream for the relatives. Frank, who now spent all of his time with the neighborhood boys, had not come, but I barely noticed. I was lost inside myself, not sure what I wanted—perhaps the stopping of time. I knew I would never see some of my classmates again, not in all the years stretching ahead of us. I wanted to say goodbye one more time, but they had all scattered, leaving for their own parties, their own lives.

I turned away from the door, the light from inside the auditorium streaming into the night, and began to walk home. A voice called out, "Lollie!" It was Uncle Karl. "Would you like a ride home?" he asked.

His car smelled of leather and smoke. He started the engine and swung out into the street, moving in and out of the pools of yellow light falling from the lamps. After we had driven several blocks in silence, he said, "It's all over."

"Yes," I whispered.

He was silent again. The warm night air drifted in through the open window and swirled his cigarette smoke around me. "It's funny," he said then. "You wait and wait for something to come, thinking it never will. And then when it does, you're not sure you want it after all."

When we arrived home, my mother said softly, "My first one is growing up." My father silently gave me the watch he had picked out for me and smiled, and my aunts and uncles handed me envelopes with five-dollar bills tucked inside. They all expected me to be happy and I pretended, yes, I was. But Uncle Karl knew how I really felt. It made all the difference.

I went away to college and fell in love with the freedom of being on my own. My mother wrote me faithfully once a week, keeping me informed on the amount of rain or snow fallen recently, her garden, and the activities of the family. "Frank loves the air force," she wrote me one week. "He says he could stay in it forever. He's such a good son—not like your cousin Jeffrey. Aunt Lydia is so upset with him. He refuses to have anything to do with Uncle Karl anymore. When Aunt Lydia asks him how he can be so rude, Jeffrey storms out of the house. Now that he can drive, he demands to use the car every night, even though he is too young to have a license. He's totally destroyed one car already. Can you believe it?"

A few more years went by. Frank came home, married, and settled in the South. I graduated from college and took a teaching position on the East Coast. My parents were left alone with Aunt Lydia and Uncle Joe, their son Jeffrey, a few other relatives, and Uncle Karl.

It was summer again. I flew back home in August for a two-week visit. The first morning my mother and I sat in the kitchen drinking coffee and covered the set topics: Frank and his wife and how they did not visit often enough, the state of health of each of the relatives, the unrelenting heat. Then she sat silently, one finger circling the top of her cup slowly, carefully. After a long while she said, "Aunt Lydia was here last Sunday. Jeffrey told her something. I don't even know if I can tell you what it is."

I looked at her, waiting. She was again gazing at her cup. "What is it?" I asked finally.

"Jeffrey had been getting drunk and driving around town like a crazy fool. One day Uncle Karl came over to their house and told Aunt Lydia she should do something about it. That night she made Jeffrey sit down after supper and listen to her. She told him how humiliated she felt that Uncle Karl had to tell her to control her own son. And like always she praised Uncle Karl. 'Why can't you be more like him?' she asked Jeffrey for probably the hundredth time. Finally Jeffrey said, 'You wouldn't always say that if you knew what Uncle Karl is *really* like.'"

"What did he mean?"

"That's the terrible part . . . I just can't believe it."

"What?"

"Jeffrey told her that—that Uncle Karl did things to him when he was little."

The air closed in around me, hot and stifling. I could not breathe. "What things?"

"Do you remember all those times Uncle Karl took Jeffrey to the stock-car races? On the way back, Uncle Karl stopped on an empty country road. At first he just sat there with Jeffrey and talked about the race. Maybe he gave him a candy bar or a bottle of soda. Then, little by little, he coaxed Jeffrey into drinking whiskey from a flask he had in the glove compartment. 'You're getting to be quite a man,' he told him. 'You're old enough to drink, to have a little fun!' Then when Jeffrey was drunk . . . the poor little boy!" She stopped, wringing her hands.

"Tell me. I want to know."

"At first it wasn't so bad. He told Jeffrey that a nice game was to look at each other's penis. There was certainly nothing wrong with that, he said. That way Jeffrey could be sure that his was just

like a man's should be. Then he started touching Jeffrey there—
and said that it was all right if Jeffrey wanted to touch him back.
Then he said everything would be easier if they took off their
clothes. Nobody would see them anyway out in the country in the
dark. Uncle Karl hugged and kissed Jeffrey and told him that he
loved him, that it was all right. Sometimes Jeffrey started to cry,
but Uncle Karl said it was the whiskey. 'You're a nice boy,' he
said. 'But you're not used to drinking. That's all. I won't tell
anyone about this.'"

"How could he? How *could* he?" I demanded. My stomach had
contracted into a hard ball and I felt as if I were going to vomit. "I
just can't believe it!"

The color had faded from my mother's face, and she sat very
still, looking at her hands. "It's the worst sin of all," she continued. "Aunt Lydia is almost in shock. When she asked Jeffrey why
he had not told her what Uncle Karl was doing all those years, his
face became twisted and he began to cry. 'How could I tell you
those things about your own *brother?*' he asked. Then he went
upstairs and closed the door."

We sat silently for a long while, the heavy stillness pressing
against us. A thick black fly, its belly bulging and creamy, droned
around and around, lighting on the table and then careening into
the moist air again. The kitchen I had known all my life, the table
and chairs where we had sat with Uncle Karl over countless cups
of coffee, were suddenly soiled, contaminated, covered with invisible decay. Nothing was as it seemed. Everything was hidden,
dark, secretly roaring toward dissolution.

My mother spoke again. "I wondered about Frank. Uncle Karl
took him along all those times. Yesterday when he called I said,
'Jeffrey told Aunt Lydia a lot of awful things about Uncle Karl.' I
still thought that maybe Jeffrey was making up everything. But
when I asked Frank if Uncle Karl ever did those things to him, he
answered, 'He tried. But I wouldn't let him. I would have nothing
to do with him after he wanted to give me whiskey. Once he tried

to kiss me, but I shoved him away and jumped out of the car.'"

"Good for him!"

"Do you think Frank is telling the truth?"

"Yes," I answered. "Remember when he wouldn't go with Uncle Karl anymore? He knew then. He was only nine or ten, but he knew."

Late that night, after my mother and I had discussed Uncle Karl long into the evening without coming any closer to making sense of anything, I asked, "You're going to tell him you know, aren't you?"

She gazed into the darkness outside the window for a long time, saying nothing. Finally she looked at me, her eyes liquid. "Aunt Lydia and I have talked about it. Neither one of us has been able to sleep just thinking about it. But we don't think we should tell him."

"They were your sons he did this to! How can you *not* tell him? He's a bastard! I never want to see him again. How *could* I? How could I ever talk to him again as if none of this had happened? How can *you?*" I turned my head quickly so she would not see the tears welling in my eyelids.

"He might kill himself," she said quietly. "That's what we think. He'll kill himself if he finds out we know."

"But what if he's still doing the same things . . . to other little boys?"

Again she looked into the darkness. "Aunt Lydia and I talked about that, too. We don't think he is. He's older now. He's a deacon in the church. It's all in the past. We mustn't tell anyone."

At the end of that week, Uncle Karl pulled into the driveway late one afternoon. "I'll be upstairs," I told my mother as he came toward the door.

"Please don't go," she pleaded. "He came to see you. I told him last week that you would be here now."

He walked into the kitchen smiling, looking like always.

"Hi, Lollie," he said. "I wanted to stop in sooner, but I've been busy. How are you?"

"Fine."

He smiled again and inhaled deeply on his cigarette. "You look fine. Just fine!"

I looked past him at the leaves brushing against the window. He and my mother began talking as if everything were the same.

When it was time to fly back to my new home on the edge of the continent, to my apartment full of light and air, I climbed into the plane gratefully. Let them live their dark, secret lives. I would have no more of it.

Several years passed. I spent my summers traveling far from home with friends. At Christmas I flew to my parents' home for two short days and spent the rest of the vacation skiing. I tried not to think about Uncle Karl. Then one day I opened a letter from my mother and read, "Your second cousin, Mattie, Grace's youngest boy, was helping Uncle Karl around his shop. Uncle Karl had told Grace how Mattie needed special attention now that his father is dead. One afternoon Mattie ran sobbing into the house and told Grace how Uncle Karl had taken down both his and Mattie's pants. White stuff squirted out of Uncle Karl's penis, Mattie said. Mattie could not stop crying again. He cried all night. I hate this more than anything. . . ."

My stomach twisted in upon itself. I knew that no one would say anything to Uncle Karl. Thank God I no longer live there, I thought, and turned to the papers I had to correct.

Another summer came. I gave in to my mother's pleas to come home and made the long trip back. The days were filled with visiting and shopping. In the evenings I talked with my father in the cool night air. On the last night of my visit, my mother and I sat down together, listening to the river frogs for some time without speaking. At last she said, "Uncle Karl has been spending a lot of time in Oregon with your cousin Claire and her family."

I looked at her sharply. "You don't think he's doing anything to their son, do you?"

"No, no, I don't think so," she said quickly. "Uncle Karl has always liked Oregon, and Claire loves to have him visit. It's so lonely there. Uncle Karl mentioned that he and little James were going on a fishing trip together in two weeks. But it's just to a lake a few miles from their farm."

When I arrived back at my apartment, I knew that I had to call Claire, but I was uneasy. While I had visited her from time to time, our lives were different, separate. We were no longer best friends. How was I to pick up the phone and tell her that our uncle was a child molester? Finally, after several failed attempts, I dialed her number and let the phone ring. "I don't know how to tell you this," I began. I could barely speak. My body was shaking. My hands felt like ice. Haltingly I recounted the history of Uncle Karl's relationships with my brother and our cousins, telling how it was kept secret, telling everything I knew.

"I'm so grateful you called," Claire assured me. "I've known in the back of my mind that something was wrong. Uncle Karl seems like a lover with James. He can't take his eyes off him. He asks to sleep in his bed. Next week they were going away together, but I won't let James go." She thanked me again. We talked about the weather. I hung up. Maybe it's over, I thought. Maybe at last it's over.

Another year passed. Claire wrote me that Uncle Karl had stopped visiting. I sighed with relief and gave all my attention to my students' papers. Then one Sunday afternoon when my apartment became too still, the quiet pressing in from all sides, I called my mother for the first time in months. "Uncle Karl is in the hospital," she said quickly. "The ambulance took him there this morning."

"What's wrong?"

"Cancer." She sighed. "All those years of smoking a pack a day.

The doctors are removing one lung tomorrow, but it may be too late. He may not live. . . ." She paused. "I can't get over it. I'm the oldest, but it's my younger brother who's dying." After I hung up, I stared at the phone for a long time. So death was calling on Uncle Karl. It seemed impossible. Whether I acknowledged him or not, he had been part of my life since that morning he stood at the screen door. How could he leave forever, just like that?

Slowly I dialed his room in the hospital. He answered the phone, his voice immediately carrying me back to all the afternoons he had sat at my mother's kitchen table drinking coffee.

"You've called," he said. "It's good to hear from you."

"Thank you . . . I'm sorry you're so ill. Are you—I mean, you must be frightened. I know I would be."

"I'm scared to death."

Damn! Why had I asked? I did not want to know about his fear. Let him keep it to himself like everything else.

He began speaking again, telling me every detail of the operation. It was the anesthesia he feared the most—the long descent into darkness, the fall into the deep well from which he might never again surface.

He stopped talking. The distance between us crackled over the telephone wires. He began to cough long and hard, as if his breath were already coming from the well. Finally he stopped, took a long, slow breath, and began again. "I want to ask you something," he said.

My hands broke out in a cold sweat. Did he find out I had called Claire? Was this why he was dying?

"Will you pray for me?" he said quietly.

This is what he wanted of me—to forgive him? How could I even begin to forgive him? I had loved him! Like a fool, I had loved the uncle I thought he was.

My throat began to ache and close. I could not breathe. I knew that, despite everything, I still loved him. I wanted him to love me to the end. It was *not* all right what he had done. It would *never* be all right. I felt he knew this but could not say what had never been spoken of, never acknowledged, never told. This was the fear that threatened to swallow him whole: that he would die in silence, unforgiven.

"Lollie?" he asked. "Are you still there?"

"Yes.... I'm sorry I didn't answer.... I ..."

"It's all right. Will you pray for me?"

"Yes, Uncle Karl. I will."

"Thank you. I appreciate it. Thanks a lot."

A few days later, he died.

BELLA MOON

"Molestation must be the most profound of all my injuries because
I have waited to the last to bring it up in therapy."

*Bella Moon (a pseudonym) was born in 1924. When she was two
years old, her father left the family. She and her brother were
initially placed in an orphanage and then in a series of foster
homes. Between the ages of three and four, her foster father repeatedly molested her. During the following year, she and her
brother lived in a different home where at mealtimes they were
stripped of their clothing, and food was thrown to them on the
floor.*

*For twenty-five years, Bella was in therapy but was unable to
deal directly with the early sexual abuse. Of her latest therapist
she says, "She helped me deal with abandonment and grief at the
early disappearance of my father, with anger that has been sub-
merged for fifty years, with the inability to ask for anything, with
the peculiar effects of institutionalization. But we never discussed
the molestation. I couldn't bring myself to talk about it."*

*However, after Bella wrote "Silence," she found that she was
able to tell her therapist about the early assaults. "Knowing that
there are others who have been molested and that a book will be
published about it," she writes, "gives me the courage to begin
dealing with it."*

*Bella is the mother of two grown children. She edits an in-
house publication and works as an activist for legislation to elimi-
nate sexism and ageism in the job market.*

She describes the narrative that follows as "a story about my true experience as a child, as seen through the eyes of an old woman (myself) who has lived a life of trauma due to early and prolonged molestation and neglect."

Silence

In the early Thirties, a little girl sat on the marble stairs of a San Francisco Victorian, watching the sunlight turn gray on the marble walls. A shadow had moved over her, although nothing was blocking the sun. She felt invaded, terrorized, and finally, paralyzed, as though the invisible shadow had stolen life from her bones as well as color from the world. With a tremendous effort, the child fixed her attention on the wall and waited an insufferable frozen moment, until the sunlight revealed once again the blue veins, the sparkling grains, of the old marble stairwell. How many times was this incident reproduced in her childhood and puberty! It became her habit to stand still and wait for the switch in her mind to transport her from a gray agony to a former calm or even happy state. She did this without knowing that she was saving her life each time, at the cost of nourishing two selves within her, each unknown to the other, each the other's mortal enemy.

An old woman stood looking down at the huddled child, and saw that she was dressed in a boy's pullover sweater, shorts, and sandals, and that her shiny brown hair was carefully cut in a Dutch bob. The old woman's heart surged with pity, divining that there was something at the top of the stairs that was a threat to the child's life. Why did she not scream out? Why did the child remain silent? Was she protecting someone?

The old woman longed to comfort her. She asked the little girl

whether she remembered something pleasant. Out of a pocket
the child drew a tattered paper, the memory of a breakfast where
a fragrant wood fire burned in the grate of a large dining room in
a private home, and twenty children from the orphanage sat
around a table and ate waffles and real maple syrup. That same
lady had given her a dollhouse complete with furniture for
Christmas. Yes, that definitely canceled out the memory of— But
why remember that any longer? As long as pain, fear, and bewil-
derment linger in the child's eyes, that is as long as we will have
to remember.

Obviously the child had been frightened into lifelong silence, not
only by the thing upstairs but by a suspicion that she had had
something to do with all of it, something sinister within herself,
an alien presence that was herself. Yes, the silence was collusion
with the adults who had violated her. She was protecting them.
Already, at age six or seven, she knew the politics of survival. In
order to survive, keep quiet, and remember—you saw it, and said
nothing; you submitted, and said nothing. You did not raise a
hand, you did not run. Above all, you do not tell your mother.
The old woman wants to clasp the child and run. But there is no
place to run to. One must stand in the sunshine and bear it.

Yes, little girl, your mother surely knows about it, because it
never would have happened if she had really wanted it stopped,
would she? She would not have put you in these houses and left
you with . . . with . . . Somehow she would have found out even if
you did not tell her, because she would have wanted to know that
it had happened; she would have asked, she would have looked,
she would have listened, she would surely have asked questions,
wouldn't she?

Somehow, child, your mother feels that what is happening is all
right. Then she must be in collusion with these others, mustn't
she? Is not this also your guilty secret—that you carry these mur-
derous suspicions about your mother? But to love what is killing

you is impossible. She cannot do it. An infernal Mitsein is spawned in the child's soul. She keeps herself free to love, and lets "the other" hate. Henceforth there shall be no communication between us; let us separate as though these horrors had never happened. By this pact, we agree to live in the child's skin, so that she may live and love her mother, protect her mother from "the other's" hate, while killing herself with small doses of a potent poison. She will forever after be free to love, and, while loving, seek love's destruction. It is intolerable, monstrous. Yet she lives; the child lives, by the grace of a switch in her mind that turns gray sunshine to yellow.

Experience Gibbs

"It's time to scream, to believe that screams are heard."

Experience Gibbs (a pseudonym), who was born in 1945, takes her name from one of the signers of the Declaration of Sentiments at the first woman's rights convention at Seneca Falls in 1848. When a friend told her of this anthology, she was able to write about her uncle's assault on her twenty-two years after it happened. "At first I resisted the idea," she says. "Then I thought I might trace my growing realization of the importance of rape in my life, perhaps by collecting entries describing moments in therapy. As I thumbed through my journals, however, this method seemed painfully distant, complex. Only clear, straightforward words could test those tentative insights."

She teaches English at a midwestern university.

1952, and Other Years

The extra bedroom leading to the sleeping porch. The table clock flanked by Thomas Jefferson, the marble-topped desk, the highboy full of grandpa's hunting pictures. The awkward closet door, jamming the door to the room: You have to open one at a time.

The closet is dark like the furniture. My tall uncle, though, has no trouble reaching into it. His long, pale arms touch the corner of the shelves, his fingers search the summer bedspreads, the camping towels and sheets, the army blankets. He extracts a bottle of whiskey, half full or less.

Does he tease me? Does he offer me a drink? He stoops close. My uncle's breath makes me sick. I remember that breath. But he is on my side. Together we resist family directions. He never tells me not to ride my bike in the rain. He never tells me to avoid black men, suspect strangers. I will not betray him. He is fifty-nine. I am seven.

——————— ———————

Is it the same time or another? Probably another, the whiskey important only in endless retrospect, a clue I should have read in the wilderness trails I tracked. A party, I think, my grandparents' house full of cousins I don't know. We eat in the sun-room on card tables while the adults sit in the dining room and argue about Joe McCarthy. Do I remember this? I remember trouble (too rowdy? food stains on my dress?), anger at my mother, loneliness.

I walk upstairs, perhaps to hide my tears. Do I meet Uncle Mack again in that room by the closet with the whiskey, does he lead me to the third floor, the attic apartment he shares with my aunt? (Their door meets that of the extra bedroom, the closet: The other two have to be closed for it to open.) Or is he upstairs already, his typing attracting me by its distance from the party? Do I open his door, climb his steep steps, turn their right angle?

——————— ———————

Focus on images. The desk. The writer would have faced the stairs. Does he try to comfort me, ask a crying child to sit in his lap? Whiskey in a bottle, in a glass on the desk, on his breath, on his lips when they meet mine. The dark heavy wooden desk. The sitting man still taller than I am standing. Our secrets. I will never tell. I know you drink and I will never tell. I love you. I love your long intricate fingers working your tiny collapsible machine, your stories of Cuba, the way you became my friend. Where is my aunt? Is she helping her mother dish out chicken and dumplings, cranking peach ice cream on the screened-in porch?

His lap, his hands rubbing my legs in sympathy. Though I will not tell, his whiskey scares me. I see I have put myself in his hands. His breath clouds my lungs. His hands are working under my skirt, under my pants. I see those long fingers pulling whiskey from the closet, I am breathing those fingers, the space between my legs stings and burns. I push against him, squirming, wriggling away. I want to throw up. It is the smell of whiskey and I will never tell just let me go now let me go.

I'm off his lap, on the floor before his chair, tangled in his legs. He's laughing, but intent. His fingers unbuckle his belt, zip open his pants. His penis looms red and swollen through his shorts. I lunge for the stairs, but he catches me, easily holding both my hands in one of his, crunching them together hard, twisting. I am four-foot-two. He is six-foot-six. From the floor, he looks even bigger.

He speaks softly, insistently. Just kiss it, kiss it. I shrink into the desk well, imagining that darkness will make me invisible, hoping he can't reach me, praying God he'll let me go, praying God my mother won't hear. I'll never tell. Just kiss it, kiss it. His legs scoop me to the front of the well. Oh, mummy, I'm sorry, I'm sorry. He holds my head in his hands. I can't breathe. I will never tell just let me go. Just kiss it, kiss it. I am throwing up it is the smell of whiskey don't break my arm. Just kiss it, kiss it. Again and again. I can't scream, I can't speak, I can't breathe. My mouth, my whole face, aches from his thrusts. I cannot see him, only huge arms, only dark brown hair around a wet red penis, pushing and pushing. I kick at the chair. I scratch his arms and skin comes off in my nails. He laughs, pressing harder, pushing his penis down my throat. Kiss it, kiss it.

——————— ———————

It is almost dark. Fireflies go off and on around the roses my
grandfather planted. The sun-room is empty of cousins, though
the lights are on. From high in the mulberry tree, I see my father
climb the stairs. A slight spring breeze rustles the evening. The
leaves twist and turn, and I tremble with them. I am not crying. I
make no sound. I listen for footsteps. My fingernails are sunk in
the tree's bark. I rub a green mulberry onto my lips, chew, and
spit it out. The sourness is soothing. When my parents call, I
know they will scold me for the bark and leaf stains on my dress.

——————— ———————

Images. Silence, unspoken fear. I imagine my parents tyrants. I
sneak down the enormous stairs of our new house, through the
hallway, the dining room, the butler's pantry, to the kitchen, take
out a carving knife, carry it cocked in my hand past the squeaking
door into my bedroom, where I hide it under my pillow until the
early morning, when I reverse the process. Again and again.
Sometimes I have to pretend I went to get a glass of water. Night
after night. I know every quick hiding place from bedroom to
drawer, every hidden space. I know there will come a time when I
will have to kill them. Then, of course, I will need the knife.

——————— ———————

I sit in the back of the room in Mrs. Ward's second-grade class. I
cannot see the blackboard. I look over Alan's shoulder, or Sher-
rie's, and memorize their problems. When I can't follow the
teacher or the class, I rock back and forth. In the secret dark well
of my desk, I raise my skirt and rub my fingers over the bump
between my legs, the bump that rises to my touch. I practice

balancing on that dangerous edge with as little movement, as little noise, as possible. Mrs. Ward asks me what I am doing, I tell her my stomach hurts. She makes me keep my hands on top of the desk. She writes notes to my parents. They take me to a specialist who asks how I feel. I lie, describing stomachaches, headaches full of explosions like fireflies in the summer night. He attaches wires to my head: Nothing happens. I see they don't know, they can't tell. My parents buy me glasses, Mrs. Ward moves my desk to the front, I get hundreds in arithmetic. But even with my hands wrapped around pencil and eraser, even with my hands spread flat and empty on the desk, I sometimes start to shake.

I am twelve. Uncle Mack is dead. With the rest of the family, I throw a spade of earth into his open grave. Just let me go I'll never tell. They are surprised I'm crying.

A child's promises, a child's rules. It has taken me twenty-two years to remember this story. I sit in my apartment on a spring evening while the rain splatters on the porch outside. Bo Diddly asks, "Who do you love? Who do you love?" I am typing in the light, I have many words at my command, but part of me crouches in the desk well, kicking, silently looking for a way out, trying not to interrupt the party, trying to disappear, trying to save myself from a man I loved. It's time to say I love myself and those who give me words that circumscribe this choking silence, who hand me back my life. It's time to own the fear in that girl's honor, it's time to break her code. It's time to scream, to believe that screams are heard. It's time to tell on Uncle Mack again and again, tell until he begs us to let him go.

PART THREE

`I trusted him`

SURVIVORS OF SEXUAL ABUSE BY FRIENDS AND ACQUAINTANCES

LOIS PHILLIPS HUDSON

"I will NEVER be less furious and bitter about the way society views rape and the infinite number of psychological rapes until *society* changes."

Lois Phillips Hudson, born in 1927, was molested several times as a child. She relates these experiences in "Why Aren't There More Creative Women?" excerpted from the article as it origi-nally appeared in Plainswoman. *In reference to the subject of her article, she writes: "At some deep, and often consciously unreach-able level,* ALL *of us fear rape and unprovoked attack, because all of us know* IT CAN HAPPEN TO ANY OF US. *And that deep fear, sup-pressed by most of us, uses an enormous amount of psychic, cre-ative energy. This fear keeps us from the simple pleasure of a solitary walk in the moonlight, or even a daytime walk in many city parks. It is on solitary walks that most of us have our 'tran-scendental moments,' our times of deep insight that result in the true poetry of the world."*

Lois is an associate professor of English at the University of Washington. She is the author of The Bones of Plenty *and* Reapers of the Dust, *as well as numerous articles and short stories. She is the mother of "two magnificent daughters."*

Why Aren't There More Creative Women?

Despite all the disagreements among various schools of psychology, there are points on which almost everyone agrees. One is that we don't know very much about what we call "the creative process," but we do know that creative insights, whether they be insights that flash a marvelous metaphor into our heads, insights that enable us to put together a story or a novel, or insights that produce scientific discoveries—all these insights arise, somehow, from our subconscious. When a writer complains of "writer's block," she or he is saying that something is interfering with whatever it is that liberates our insights from our subconscious.

Now let us look at what happens to the subconscious of just about every single human female in any time, any culture. Every one of us knows that we are at the mercy of just about every physically normal male between the ages of thirteen and seventy-five. We may not let ourselves think about it, as numbers of young women who hitchhike have said to me. But it is always there—that knowledge we have had since we were very young.

And many of us have had terrible experiences by the time we are ten years old. My first was at nine. A seventy-year-old man who was the father of my mother's best friend. He was also a preacher. I had been taught to revere him. Mr. Betts did not rape me. He followed me into the woods when I thought I was alone, and he fondled me. I cannot describe my terror—not even today. Nor can I describe my feelings of guilt. I must have somehow done something hideously wrong, out exploring alone in the woods when he came upon me. Otherwise, how could a preacher, the father of my mother's beloved friend, how could he have done that?

And what was it that was wrong with me?

When I was thirteen, my mother arranged for me to catch a ride, with our neighbor, to town six miles away. It was during the war, and we had gas rationing. I was to ride to Kirkland with Mr. Ahmann, go to the dentist, and wait for my father to pick me up there on his way home from work at Boeing. Mr. Ahmann, the father of thirteen children, including three girls who were my best friends, took a back route through what was at that time a forest. He stopped the car and turned to me with a look in his eyes that, again, I cannot describe. He pulled me to him, his hand over my new breasts, kissed me with his tongue in my mouth. I had never been kissed in my life by anybody except my mother. (Mr. Ahmann, incidentally, is one of the reasons why, three years later, I didn't date boys, to the consternation of my concerned guidance counselor.) He was trembling, but for the first time in my life, I really understood all the implications of male strength. I was an unusually strong, athletic girl, and I had my full growth, but I knew I was helpless. Even so, I thought of how I could manage to break away and run into the forest. No, I thought. He can catch you. It's better to beg.

So I begged. What does it do to a human female to have to beg for her survival—her plain, simple physical survival—from the time she is ten years old? Or even younger. What does it do to us to be taught to beg, to flatter, to cajole, taught by both men and women, from the time we are tiny? I'm not talking about optimum conditions for creativity here. I'm talking about survival—physical survival. What does this do to our sense of ourselves as creative human beings? I submit that the creative woman has surmounted obstacles that most men have never imagined. I begged him. I made my self into nothing, and begged.

And after a few more agonizing squeezings of new tender breasts, and a few more kisses with his disgusting saliva all over my face, he stopped trembling and let me go. In a shaky voice, he told me he would let me go if I promised never to tell anybody. Of course I promised. So far as I can remember, that was the first time I made a promise I knew I didn't intend to keep. (Oh, yes,

we women are so sly and cunning.) That was the first time my
adult integrity was raped.

I did, finally, after I recovered from the worst of my own self-
loathing, after I had scrubbed my mouth so many times that it no
longer felt so filthy that I couldn't speak of it—I did finally tell my
mother. I knew it would hurt her, but I had to. And I must insert
here, How many girls *can't* tell their mothers? How many girls
have mothers who have been so frightened by men that they
have, in subtle ways, made it clear that they do not want to hear
any such stories from their daughters?

And when I think of my father at that time, I am nauseated.
Every time the Ahmann girls came over to our house, he had to
get his hands on them. There was always a funny, laughing reason
to give them a hug. (He never, of course, hugged me!) Always a
reason to whistle at them, pinch them, slap their fannies, as the
male saying goes. I know that my father would never have done
more than that, but I could tell they hated it. And I knew how
they would feel if they ever knew what their father had done to
me!

So—we never tell, do we?

But we need our egos. At a cocktail party for me as an author, a
man I knew fairly well, a colleague of my husband's, said to me,
with the greatest of admiration, "Lois, I can't imagine how much
guts it takes to be a writer. You must have to have the ego of a
prizefighter." I agreed. You have to have an ego that will make
you get up again, no matter how many times you've been
knocked down. To do anything creative—in science, in business,
anything—you have to get up again and try again. So who are we?
If we have no right to our own bodies, how can we have the right
to our own wills? (It's hard to have the ego of a prizefighter when
you know that any punk kid may take a notion to rape and perhaps kill you.) And, most of all, there is our feeling that we don't
have the right to our own feelings.

I think the belief that one has the right to her own feelings has got to be the basis of any creativity. You have to feel that what you see, what you hear, what you think—that these things are totally valid.

But what if you are told, in a thousand ways, from the time that you are born, that you can and will be raped? What if you are told that whether you want sex or not, whether you want to cater to another person's ego or not, this is what you were put on earth to do? What rights do you have then? How do you dare to have your own feelings? What great artist does not express his or her own feelings?

What, besides the right to her own feelings, does any creative person have to feel? You have to feel that you are in control. This is a story, this is an essay, this is a novel, this is a painting, this is a musical composition that I will control! This is what I want to say, and I will say it!

If you are a human female, somehow you have to decide that you do have a right to your own feelings, a right to control what you are doing, and that despite everything that everybody has taught you, you will assert that right.

HONOR MOORE

"The prosecuting attorney said to Joan Little, referring to her rape by the guard whom she later stabbed, 'What, you didn't holler? You didn't shout? You didn't fight him off?' I remembered my feelings of powerlessness and began this poem."

Honor Moore was born in 1945. When she was four years old, her parents moved to Jersey City, New Jersey, where her father, an Episcopal priest, became part of an experimental ministry at an inner-city church. Both her parents believed that the family should be part of the community to which they ministered, and modeled themselves after the French worker-priests. Honor describes their life at this time as one of contradictions: "Our house was open. There was always hot soup on the stove for anyone who came to the door hungry, clothes in the basement for those whose apartments burned, for the derelict who sold the coat he'd worn last week for a bottle of Sneaky Pete. A young man who also baby-sat for us pawned the church's typewriter and mimeograph machine and was arrested."

The events described in "First Time: 1950" happened when Honor was five years old. She remained silent, afraid that the young man, who was part of the community, would go to jail if she told. As she grew older, Honor felt that perhaps she had in some way provoked the abuse. Her feelings of shame about the incident continued into adulthood and interfered with her sexual relationships until she was able to break her silence.

She began the poem when Joan Little was on trial, but it remained an unfocused rough draft until she was working on sestinas at a writers' retreat: "A man violently insulted me, and I again

172

*felt enraged and powerless. I went straight to my studio, pulled
out the material, and wrote it in sestina form."*

The poem was first published in Shenandoah: The Washington and Lee University Review. *Honor has published many other
poems and has completed a first collection. A verse play about
her mother's death,* Mourning Pictures, *was published in* The
New Women's Theatre: Ten Plays by Contemporary American
Women *(Vintage, 1977), which she edited. Currently she is working on a biography of her grandmother, Margarett Sargent, who
gave up a successful career as a painter at the age of forty-five.*

Honor Moore's most recent book is Memoir, *published in
1988.*

First Time: 1950

In the back bedroom, laughing when you pull
something fawn-colored from your black
tight pants, the unzipped chino slit.
I keep myself looking at the big belt
buckled right at my eyes, feel the hand
riffle my hair: You are called Mouse, baby-

sitter trusted Wednesdays with my baby
brother. With me. I still see you pull
that huge bunch of keys from a pocket, hand
them to my brother, hear squeaking out back
Mrs. Fitz's clothesline as you unbelt,
turn me to you, my face to the open slit.

It's your skin, this thing, head, its tiny slit
like the closed eye of a still-forming baby:
As you stroke, it stiffens like a new belt—

your face gets almost sick. I want to pull
away, but you grip my arm: I tell by your black
eyes you won't let go. With your left hand

you take my chin. With your other hand
you guide it, head reddening, into my slit,
my five-year-old mouth. In the tight black
quiet of my shut eyes, I hear my baby
brother shaking the keys. You lurch, pull
at my hair. I don't breathe, feel buckle, belt,

pant. It tastes lemony, musty as a belt
after a day of sweat. Mouth hurts, my hands
push, push at your hips. I gag. You let me pull
free. I open my eyes, see the strange slits
yours are; you don't look at me. "Babe, babee—"
You are moaning, almost crying. The black

makes your skin clam-white now, your jewel-black
eyes blacker. You buckle up the thick belt.
When you take back the keys, my baby
brother cries. You extend a shaking hand
you make kind. In daylight through the wide slit
an open shade leaves, I see her pull,

Mrs. Fitz pulling in her rusty, soot-black
line. Framed by the slit, her window, her large hands
flash, sort belts, dresses, shirts, baby clothes.

BILLIE HOLIDAY

"My God, it's terrible what something like this does to you. It takes years and years to get over it; it haunts you and haunts you."

"Lady Day" was born Eleanora Fagan in Baltimore, Maryland, on April 7, 1915. In 1928 she and her mother moved to New York City, where she was inspired by recordings of Louis Armstrong and Bessie Smith. At the age of fifteen, she began to sing professionally in a Harlem nightclub. In 1933 she made her first recording, with Benny Goodman.

During the Forties she became well known for the unique, bittersweet quality of her voice, her striking beauty, and the gardenia she usually wore in her hair. After 1950, drug addiction increasingly affected her health and career. She died in New York City on July 17, 1959, at the age of forty-four. The piece reprinted here, and the epigraph above, are excerpted from her autobiography.

from Lady Sings the Blues

One day when I came home from school, Mom was at the hairdresser's and there was nobody in the house but Mr. Dick, one of our neighbors. He told me Mother had asked him to wait for me and then take me a few blocks away to somebody's house, where she would meet us.

175

Without me thinking anything about it, he took me by the hand and I went along. When we got to the house, a woman let us in. I asked for my mother and they said she would be along soon. I think they told me she had called them on the telephone and said she would be late. It got later and later and I began to get sleepy. Mr. Dick saw me dozing and took me into a back bedroom to lie down. I was almost asleep when Mr. Dick crawled up on me and started trying to do what my cousin Henry used to try. I started to kick and scream like crazy. When I did, the woman of the house came in and tried to hold my head and arms down on the bed so he could get at me. I gave both of them a hard time, kicking and scratching and screaming. Suddenly, when I was catching my breath, I heard some more hollering and shouting. The next thing I knew, my mother and a policeman broke the door down. I'll never forget that night. Even if you're a whore, you don't want to be raped. A bitch can turn twenty-five hundred tricks a day and she still don't want nobody to rape her. It's the worst thing that can happen to a woman. And here it was happening to me when I was ten.

I couldn't figure out how my mother had managed to find where they had taken me. But when she had come home, one of Mr. Dick's girl friends, a jealous hustler, was waiting on the porch. She warned Mom to keep me away from her man.

Mom tried to brush her off, telling her I was just a kid and to quit being jealous and silly.

"Just a kid?" said this hustler, laughing. "She ran off with my man. She's with him right now, and if you don't believe me I'll tell you where you'll find them."

Mom didn't waste no time. She called the police and took this jealous bitch by the arm and dragged her to the house where they had me. And a house it was, too.

But that wasn't the worst of it. The cops dragged Dick off to the police precinct. I was crying and bleeding in my mother's arms, but they made us come along too.

When we got there, instead of treating me and Mom like some-body who called the cops for help, they treated me like I'd killed somebody. They wouldn't let my mother take me home. Mr. Dick was in his forties, and I was only ten. Maybe the police sergeant took one look at my breasts and limbs and figured my age from that, I don't know. Anyway, I guess they had me figured for having enticed this old goat into the whorehouse or some-thing. All I know for sure is they threw me into a cell. My mother cried and screamed and pleaded, but they just put her out of the jailhouse and turned me over to a fat white matron. When she saw I was still bleeding, she felt sorry for me and gave me a couple glasses of milk. But nobody else did anything for me ex-cept give me filthy dirty looks and snicker to themselves.

After a couple of days in a cell they dragged me into court. Mr. Dick got sentenced to five years. They sentenced me to a Catho-lic institution.

*   *   *

Things had happened to me that no amount of time could change or heal. I had gone to jail when I was ten because a forty-year-old man had tried to rape me. Sure, they had no more business put-ting me in that Catholic institution than if I'd been hit by a damn truck. But they did. Sure, they had no business punishing me, but they had. For years I used to dream about it and wake up holler-ing and screaming. My God, it's terrible what something like this does to you. It takes years and years to get over it; it haunts you and haunts you.

Getting booked and busted again didn't help, either. I might explain the first rap was a freak accident. But the second was tougher. For years it made me feel like a damn cripple. It changed the way I looked at everything and everybody. There was one chance I couldn't take. I couldn't stand any man who didn't know about the things that had happened to me when I was a kid. And I was leery of any man who could throw those things back at me in a quarrel. I could take almost anything, but, my God, not that. I didn't want anyone around who might ever hold this over me or even hint that on account of it he was a cut above me.

KAREN ASHERAH

"Somehow I deadened the experience by years of denying that it happened. To tell about it is to finally gain my sense of power. I am angry!"

Karen Asherah was born in 1950 in a coastal town in California. After the molestation experiences described in "Daddy Kanagy," Karen rebelled daily against returning to the child-care center where the incidents occurred. "I didn't tell my mother why I didn't want to go," she writes. "I didn't know why myself.... I also felt at the time that being abused sexually was normal somehow, something I could just expect as a child."

It was as she grew into adulthood that Karen realized the implications of the molestations: "The overall influence of Daddy Kanagy as well as other adult figures of power in my life was tremendous. Now I can see that I gave my power away ... I didn't say no to the molester or tell my mother. I didn't trust myself. It is still hard to trust myself, to take hold of what I want and do it."

Daddy Kanagy

When I was eight, my mother got a job in another town and my family moved. My two brothers and I were dropped off mornings at a child-care center.

The center was run by an old retired couple, the Kanagys. Mrs.

Kanagy did most of the chores and took care of the children. "Daddy" Kanagy, as everyone affectionately called him, sat around, watched TV, and sometimes amused the children. Mrs. Kanagy looked after him, as he was older than she and approaching senility.

There was a big mulberry tree in the backyard with a tree fort, a hammock, and a summerhouse for picnics. The swing set and slide were to the side of the yard at the edge of a big field where we played and ran. I can remember good times, making mulberry hamburgers and watching Mickey Mouse and Popeye cartoons in the playroom with the other children. Sometimes Mrs. Kanagy gave us ice-cream cones in the afternoon. And there was a talking parakeet that ate breakfast on Daddy Kanagy's shoulder.

I was a shy child and hated to have to talk in front of the class. In second grade, the teacher asked us to tell the class about our fathers. Having never met my father, I didn't know what to say. Although I knew his name and occupation, I could feel the blood rushing to my cheeks. I always felt odd because I never had a dad.

So when I started going to the Kanagys before and after school, I was enthralled with the idea of having a daddy. My mother, hoping as I did that he could fulfill the father role, praised him to me, always telling me how special and kind he was. Our needs for a daddy were so strong that I tried to ignore the events that followed.

At first I was simply confused and hurt—like the day a boy put his finger into a hole in my pants. I ran to Daddy Kanagy for consolation and protection. His response was a grin and a chuckle.

Then one afternoon when I was just waking up from a nap, he sat next to me on the side of the bed. He put his big heavy fingers in my pants and began rubbing my clitoris. I had no idea what he was trying to do. He asked, yet sort of told me, "It feels good, doesn't it?" All I knew was I couldn't say no. I felt powerless to move. I said Yes. Then Mrs. Kanagy walked into the room. She stood there, stunned, and finally told me to go out and play. Afterward she never mentioned this episode to me. And I never mentioned it to her. It was our secret.

The incidents continued. I was sitting in the back seat of the Kanagys' car, my knees bent up against the seat ahead. Mrs. Kanagy had gone to shop and Daddy Kanagy reached back and put his hand on my genitals. He told me never to tell anyone. But I already knew I wouldn't say a word. My mother adored him, idealized him, and I felt I needed to protect our image of our great Daddy.

Although I never expressed the wariness I had for Daddy Kanagy, I became convinced that grown men, especially daddies, were not to be trusted. Walking to school one day in the rain, the father of a classmate offered me a ride, but I refused. He kept saying, "Don't you remember me? I'm so-and-so's father." But I just repeated my refusal. Another time, standing with other children at the bus stop, they all got into a car driven by someone's father, except me.

Ironically, "Father Knows Best" was one of my favorite TV programs, but in real life I have grown up trusting few fathers or even the concept of a good father.

It wasn't until we had moved to another town, years had gone by, and Daddy Kanagy had died that I told my mother. She was outraged. All she could say was "Why didn't you tell me?" She has never understood why I kept silent.

Many years later, I told my friend and lover about the incident. It was like a ghost returning as the familiar grin came to his face and he said, "You must have been a sexy little girl."

NAOMI SCHWARTZ

"Through therapy and talking with friends, I learned to feel compassion rather than contempt for the needy, small self I was."

Naomi Schwartz was born in 1950. When she was small, her father left the family, and she felt deserted. Her poem, "Peaches of My Childhood," was written about a molestation that occurred shortly after her father's departure. "I think my poem is accurate in depicting the attractions of the forbidden when a child is abandoned by a parent," she writes, "... the combined sense of 'wrongness' and need."

Naomi has managed both a housecleaning business and an antique store and continues to write, looking for new perspectives about her life.

The Peaches of My Childhood

The peaches of my childhood
took two hands to hold.
Patsy, the Italian grocer,
handed me that deep escape
starting from his huge palm.
Then patted me, rough skin catching
in hair strands fallen in my eye.
My hasty first bite brought on

his laughter. Patsy swelled with
pleasure at my pleasure.

O Patsy, you make me remember my father;
he and I arm-in-arm
come to ask you for tomatoes, cucumbers
crisp lettuce.

Now the center fallen out;
father gone . . . mother comes home
alone to a heavy ragged sleep.
Her navy-blue room is all ocean
and no air. Light has no place
in the blue dark my father wants
no part of.

She will push away his presence.
She will paint the room white.

——————— ———————

The housepainter arrives warm and dark
with fingers thick as my father's
that used to bend paper into airplanes
and work cloth napkins into white roses.

A big man again moves in our house, his rollers
erase the gray departure in cleaned out drawers.
He is painting the inside
of my mother's closet
and invites me to help.
I squeeze into the dark
press close and grasp

the roller with both hands
glad to be of use.

Fitting his big hands
under my arms; my breath
is trapped.
I remember this moment—
new and not new.
I wish the housekeeper's strident
voice would gather me
into its clear sharp lines.

The white paint spreads easily.
I do   I don't want to pull away.
The buzz in my ears grows
steadily louder.
I know this burning must be a secret.
He is on his knees now   breath ragged—
it's going too far into what
I don't know
and I say, "I'm tired"
and know I'll return.

MIRIAM MONASCH

"I would like to have a child as soon as I feel I can raise her or him not to be a victim. I'm not there yet, but I've come a long way. I have faith in myself."

Miriam Monasch was born on November 10, 1952. When she was a child, her family moved often, averaging two and a half years in various cities in California, the Midwest, and Europe. "My mother," Miriam writes, "claims I was always a happy child. I think it was around the time of the events in this story that I stopped trusting the perceptions other people have of me."

"The Fourth of July" recounts one incident in a series of molestations that happened to Miriam as a young girl. She told no one about these experiences and as an adolescent completely blocked the memory of them. However, their effects on her were deep: "The nightmares, the feelings of guilt about everything, and the definition of myself, first and foremost, in sexual terms were the unconscious outcome. By the time I reached adulthood, my sexuality . . . consumed me. But it could never be satisfied, because it had, quite literally, been perverted. My innocence revolted against it. And it was this battle between opposing parts of myself which made my life intolerable."

The pain and confusion of not being able to maintain any lasting relationships led Miriam to seek help. With the aid of therapists, she has been able to uncover the source of this pain. "It is an ongoing process," she says.

Miriam acts, sings, and writes in the lesbian community in Minneapolis. She has written a semiautobiographical one-act play about *child sexual abuse and the attempt to deny that pain through the abuse of chemicals. "Each time I perform it," she states, "I go through the stages of remembering—through pain, to anger, and finally, absolution."*

The Fourth of July

There is always jazz music when we go to the Jeffersons' house. Mr. Jefferson is a musician. He plays saxophone in a little band that plays in bars. Mrs. Jefferson gets a job as a cocktail waitress wherever the band works. My father says it's because she's so jealous, and he laughs. My mother laughs at that, too. She doesn't know what it feels like not to trust your husband.

Brad Jefferson is my brother's best friend. They are in the same scout troop. He is tall and thin. Michael isn't. But they both wear glasses. Brad is okay.

The Jeffersons have a big Doughboy swimming pool in their backyard. It fills almost the whole yard except the patio where the barbecue is. They ask us all to come over for a picnic sometimes and we go swimming. I used to like to go to the Jeffersons' to go swimming, but I don't like to anymore. I don't like Greg Jefferson, Brad's big brother.

But today is the Fourth of July and we are going to the Jeffersons' house. This time there will be fireworks and more people. The band is going to play on the patio instead of records. Maybe that will make it different.

Michael and I sit in the back seat and my father drives. My mother is just learning how to drive, but she doesn't like to. She says she likes to just relax and look out the window and not worry, but she can't do that if she's driving. I sit behind my father way back in the seat and right next to the door. I don't even want to look out the window. My mother is leaning her head on one arm.

Her hair is blowing in the wind. She is wearing the sunglasses with the plaid frames. Michael is bouncing up and down on the seat till my father has to turn around and tell him to knock it off. Then he says, "How's my little dummy?" and smiles at me in the mirror.

I say, "Okay."

When we get to the Jeffersons', there are already people there. We're still the only kids. There are hamburgers and hot dogs on the grill, and corn wrapped in tinfoil right on the coals. Brad and Greg are in the pool. Michael goes right into the house to put on his suit, and I go with him. I wait outside the bathroom door and ask him to hurry up. I know Greg is swimming. When Michael comes out, I go right in and lock the door. I put on my swimsuit very fast. Then I open the door and run back outside. Greg is still in the pool. He and Brad are fighting over a green rubber raft. He is holding Brad under the water for a long time, but then he lets him come up. He is a lot bigger and heavier than Brad. Michael goes into the water. I go and sit on my mother's lap. She is talking to Mrs. Jefferson and another lady. They both have tall, thin glasses with straws in them. My mother's glass is shorter with lots of ice. That seems right because Mrs. Jefferson is a lot taller than my mother or her husband or almost anybody. She always wears high heels, too. She has very red hair and a little bracelet around her ankle.

My mother tells me to go into the pool. I don't say anything. I just stay right there. The other lady smiles at me. She has brown curly hair that is very shiny. She is wearing a shirt with bright pink flowers on it and shorts. She looks like she comes from Hawaii. My mother lifts me off her lap and says, "Go on and play with the boys before they get tired and come out." She won't let me go into the pool alone. It is too deep for me.

I climb up the ladder and let myself down into the pool. It's not too cold. Hanging on to the side, I let myself go all the way under to get my hair wet. I like the way it looks when it's wet. It's straight and smooth against my head almost. The boys are on the other side of the pool. I hold on to the rim and kick my legs.

All of a sudden there are hands around my waist from underneath. I kick harder, but Greg is lifting me up into the air. I am kicking as hard as I can, but he is holding me up away from him. Everyone is laughing. I see my father standing by the barbecue looking over and laughing. Then Greg drops me into the water. I touch bottom. I kick and move my arms around in big circles to get to the top again. Greg grabs my wrist and pulls me to the surface. My hair is like a wet blanket on my face and I am gasping for air. He guides my hand to the rail. He lets go of me and dips back underwater. I feel a hand between my legs. I kick hard again and he is gone.

No one is in the pool anymore. It is getting dark. I am waiting for a hamburger to get done for me. I am standing next to the grill watching it. It smells juicy and smoky at the same time. My bathing suit is still wet. I have my towel wrapped around my shoulders, but I'm shivering a little even by the fire. I have to go to the bathroom, too. But I don't want to go in the house. The boys are in there. My mother sees that I am cold and tells me to go into the house and put some dry clothes on. I look right at her for a long time until she says, "This minute." I go up to her and ask her if she will come with me. She laughs and tells me that I'm too old to need help dressing. I turn and walk toward the house. It is almost dark now. The band has gotten all their instruments out. Some people are laughing and making jokes. Almost everybody is having a good time.

I walk through the house slowly. I can hear the boys in Brad's room watching TV and talking. Greg is the loudest. I walk very softly and don't make any noise. I go in the bathroom and lock the door before I turn the light on. It is hard getting my bathing suit off because it's so cold and wet. I am goose-pimply all over. I look over to the hamper where I left my clothes, but they're not there. I look inside the hamper. They aren't anywhere. I don't know who took them but I know that I have to go and find them. I look at my suit rolled up on the floor. I can't put that back on. So I wrap my towel all around me. I unlock the door and open it as quietly as I can. I peek out into the hall. The voices are still loud a few doors down and the party noise comes in from the backyard. I go into the living room where my mother had left her beach bag. My clothes are lying on top of it. They are practically the only things in the room that aren't black or white or dark red. Before we met the Jeffersons, I didn't know anyone who painted their living room black.

I start back to the bathroom as quickly as I can go and not make any noise. I am almost at the door when it opens wide from the inside. Greg says, "Come on in, I'll be through in a minute."

I don't move.

Then he says, "Hurry up. Get in here."

I walk in clutching my clothes in front of me. He closes the door and locks it. I stand in the corner next to the hamper. He stands by the toilet, kind of smiling over at me. He unzips his pants and takes out his penis. He holds it like my father and Michael do when they are going to the bathroom. But nothing comes out. He starts to move his hand and rub it. He is still smiling at me. His penis gets bigger and stiffer. He says, almost in a whisper, "Come here. Don't you want to touch it? Touch it."

I don't want to move.

He stops smiling and says, "Come here."

I walk over to the toilet. He reaches out and takes my clothes out of my hands and throws them across the room onto the floor. He pulls the towel away from me. He takes my wrist and puts my hand on his penis. He says, "Hold on to it and rub it up and down." Both his hands are holding me by the shoulders. I am standing right in front of him and his penis is right in front of my face. I do what he says to do.

Soon he starts to breathe heavier. I look up at his face and see that he has closed his eyes. His big fingers are kneading into my back. He sighs a little and then says quickly, "Kiss it." He has never said that before and I look up at him. He is looking down at me again, but he isn't smiling anymore. "Go on. Kiss it." With one hand behind my neck, he pulls my head toward his penis. I purse my lips and touch the end of it. He takes my head between his hands and pushes against my face. "Open your mouth," he says, but I pretend that I don't hear him because his hands are over my ears. He bends over me and repeats it. I open my mouth and he pushes his penis into it. It is big and fills my whole mouth. I have to stretch my jaws as wide as I can and it hurts. He pulls back and forth and tries to push deeper, faster and faster. Then, before I know what's happening, he pulls away from me and turns and stands over the toilet again. I think he is going to the bathroom, but it comes out differently. The air is passing through his teeth very slowly.

He says, "Hurry up and get dressed." I can hear the music outside now. He tucks his penis in his pants and zips himself up. He sits on the edge of the bathtub and watches me put my shorts and T-shirt on. When I have all my clothes on, he says, "Go on outside. I'll be right out." He unlocks the door and I go out.

I walk out the back door and stand on the porch. Michael and Brad are eating hamburgers at the picnic table. Mr. Jefferson is playing his saxophone and the other men in the band are playing along. Mrs. Jefferson is mixing another drink in her tall, thin glass. My mother and father are dancing. They hold each other and swing around to the music. He spins her around very fast and she laughs. They see me and smile at me. My mother says, "Your hamburger is on the table. It's getting cold." They keep dancing.

I go to the picnic table and sit down across from Michael and Brad. They act like they don't see me and whisper to each other. I am sitting still and staring at my hamburger. I can't eat it. I don't know what to do. I just sit and stare.

BEVERLY SKY

"I felt like I could trust the priest. The idea that I could not never even occurred to me."

Beverly Sky was born in Salzburg, Austria, in 1947 to a Jewish mother and a Roman Catholic father. After the family immigrated to the United States, Beverly's mother annually burned a candle in a glass bearing the Star of David in memory of her parents. In all other aspects she gave up Judaism and raised her children as devout Roman Catholics. While Beverly's father did not attend mass regularly, he believed that his children should be observant Catholics and once told Beverly that she should become either a nun or a nurse when she was grown.

The initial effect on Beverly of the incident described in "The Priest's Kiss" was a loss of faith in the saintliness of the clergy. She also felt guilty for what happened, as if somehow it had been her fault. "After that I was no longer 'daddy's girl' as I had been in the past," she writes. "There was a distance between us that could never be bridged."

Several years after the incident, Beverly joined a youth group in a Jewish community center in her neighborhood. "I was attracted to the idea," she says, "that there is no intermediary between God and me." She lives in Boston with her two children and works full-time as a graphic designer.

A Priest's Kiss

It was Ash Wednesday, 1957. I was ten years old. Because I had an ear infection, I had to go to a special clinic during the time of normal church services. I arranged with the priest to come to church at 7:30 in the morning to receive the blessing and the ash on my forehead.

The priest was in his early thirties, quiet, soft-spoken, and to my eyes, handsome. Once before during confession the honey-combed screen began to spin, the cubicle began to feel close. I can still remember the smell of incense and musty red curtains as I fainted. The next thing I knew, the priest was carrying me outside to get some air. I sat on a wooden folding chair and he offered me a glass of water that I imagined tasted like holy water.

That morning he greeted me at the door of the church, and as we walked down the aisle, I noticed the lights were off. There was no one else in the church at that hour. It was eerie and dim as he led me to the vestibule to the left of the altar where the ashes were kept. Light came through the stained-glass windows that were partially covered by red velvet curtains. Rows of black and purple cassocks, vestments, and books lined the walls. He didn't turn on the light. He brought forth a small kneeling stand and I knelt down. As he rubbed my forehead and recited the blessing, I clasped my hands together in prayer. When I opened my eyes, he was lifting me up into a tight embrace and kissing me on the mouth. I was shocked and terrified, but I didn't want to seem afraid. I thanked him, and left quickly.

I went to the clinic, and by the time I came home I had resolved not to tell my father what had happened. I didn't think he'd believe me anyway. How could I prove it? I do not recall if I told my mother, but I doubt it. I announced several days later that I would not go to church again. My father asked me why, and I replied that since he did not attend church, I would not. Since he worked weekends at the time, the discussion ended there. He did not speak to me for two years after that. I preferred to suffer his "disappointment" in me rather than face the possible humiliation of confrontation with my father.

I did not set foot in a church again until I was nineteen, and then only to admire the architecture.

JANA VINCENTI

"My mom wrote this down while I told her. I didn't want to think about my rape by myself."

Jana Vincenti (a pseudonym) was born in 1966 in Berkeley, California. At the age of seven, she was raped. While she could not tell her mother about the assault then, she was able to tell her four years later. Her mother, Arlene, reacted with shock and horror, not only because her daughter had been raped but because she herself had a history of child sexual abuse. As a child Arlene had been repeatedly molested by family friends, and when she was fifteen years old, she was kidnapped and raped. Jana was born of this rape.

Arlene has encouraged Jana to keep talking about the experience. "I tell her that rape has long been a tactic used by men to suppress women," Arlene writes. "We both find great strength in being able to share these common experiences with each other as women."

At age 17, Jana felt that the experience caused her to think differently from other girls her age about being a woman. "I'm only four feet and eleven inches, but I'm big on how to defend myself," she states. "My mom took me to self-defense classes. I think women should be strong!"

Daughter

When I was seven years old, a man who was about thirty raped me. He was my mother's boyfriend. I didn't understand what was happening to me then, but now that I am almost thirteen years old, I do.

It all started when my mother's boyfriend came over to visit her and she was in the shower. I was in my T-shirt and under-wear, which were kind of holey on the bottom. Freddie noticed and stuck his finger up my vagina and it hurt. I said, "Quit!" and pushed him away. He did it again and then he quit.

Then Freddie went into my mom's bedroom and started strip-ping off his pants and shirt. He pulled down his underwear a little. I passed by the bathroom and said goodnight to my mom. Then I went to the door of my mom's bedroom and said good-night to Freddie. Freddie told me to come into the bedroom to get a dollar he had for me in his hand. I stayed in the doorway, afraid; I thought he would try to put his finger in my underwear again. I told him my mother had told me never to take money from people unless she was there. He stretched out on the bed and leaned toward me, grabbed my hand, and pulled me into the bedroom. Then he said, "I'll give you a dollar if you touch this." He was holding his penis in his hand. It was big and looked hard. I was very scared and backed into my mother's closet. He told me to come out of the closet. By now he was sitting on the edge of my mom's bed, still holding his penis. Thick, clear white sticky stuff was coming out of it. He said, "Let me put my penis in your vagina and I'll give you a dollar."

I tried to run out of the room, but he grabbed my hands and pulled me real close to him and took down my underwear. Then he pulled me on top of him and grabbed my bum and rubbed his penis between my legs, holding me by my bum. I felt sticky stuff all over me and it hurt real bad. I don't know if his penis went in, but it felt like it did—like something was stretching down there.

My vagina hurt for three days afterward. It was all red and swollen. I showed my mom because I was real worried and she wondered what I had been doing. I was afraid to tell her what Freddie had done because I didn't know what had happened to my vagina, whether or not it had been injured.

Now that I am older, I wish Freddie would be thrown in jail for what he did to me, or his penis cut off since he doesn't know how to use it. Grown men shouldn't be allowed to go around hurting little girls with their penises.

LILLIAN KELLY

"Aside from the fear, confusion, and shame, the molestation was as if I'd passed through an enormous threshold, as big as birth."

Lillian Kelly was born in 1947 in Marin County, California. As a young adolescent, she was molested by the father of a friend. She told no one. Soon after this incident, she began to overeat and was obese throughout high school and college. While she developed a few close female friendships, she did not form any relationships with males for a number of years.

Lillian's molestation experience was life-changing: "It created a new person where the old one had been," she writes. She is grateful that it was brief, never repeated, and did not involve a family member. "I was then, as I am now, thankful for the warning," she explains, "even as I was and am thankless for the fear."

She illustrates the effects of the experience with an allegory:

Some years after (it's always "before" and "after," isn't it?), during my senior year of high school, my close friend received two antique vases in the mail. One arrived whole, the other hopelessly shattered. My friend labored, sometimes passionately, sometimes indifferently, all through that year piecing together the delicate porcelain. When her cat knocked the half-completed reconstruction from her desk, breaking it in new places, I think my friend saw it as a minor and interesting setback, while I despaired.

She completed the project, but the vase she produced could hardly be called complete. Tiny and large chips, once part of the original, had inevitably been lost, hidden in the packing material, or carried away by a little sister. This vase was more a product of my friend's labor than that of the original artist.

Strangely, though, the new vase, for all its disfigurement, scars, chips, and ragged lip, for all the horror of the shattering and an imperfect mending, when set beside its unblemished twin, was the more splendid of the two.

My friend presented her vase to me as a graduation gift, and I have it still.

Aftermath

Sometimes,
When my lover breathes a certain
     way
In his passion,
My heart goes cold,
My mind goes dark.
I wait, silently.

Sometimes,
When my daughter rushes to her
     games,
Carelessly, singing,
I call her back
And speak and speak
The unnamed fear.

PART FOUR

"I never saw him before"

SURVIVORS OF SEXUAL ABUSE BY STRANGERS

JADE GATES

"Finally now I can say about the sexual assaults, "I am innocent," and believe it."

Jade Gates was born in the early Fifties in Long Beach, California. At the age of seventeen, she ran away from home to the Haight-Ashbury district of San Francisco. By the time she was twenty-one, she was divorced and the mother of two small children. For the next six years, she raised her children alone.

Several years ago in a women's writing workshop led by Ellen Bass, she heard Ellen read a poem about innocence. Shortly thereafter she wrote "And Now."

Jade has remarried and attended college. Although she feels that she was traumatized by the sexual assaults she suffered as a child, she does not think they left permanent scars. "I was young," she writes. "Those things happened. I shivered and sometimes cried, but then it was over. I took the memories and stored them away with others, like when I stole a yellow balloon from Long's Drug Store and the day I peed in Margaret's backyard."

And Now

And now, now that you have told me I am innocent, told me plainly, clearly, several times, I can remember, remember so much more. My childhood flashes in front of me like a labyrinth with an exposed penis at every corner. All these incidents happened before I was fourteen and I never told anyone.

There was the man who stopped in front of my house while I was playing ballerina on the lawn, twirling in my mother's soft pink dress. Getting out of his car, he asked if I wanted a ride. I ran into the house and shook behind the locked door.

There was the man who slowly followed me in his shiny green car as I walked home from school. When I hurried my pace, he drove faster, until finally I hopped a fence and darted through some unknown backyards.

There was a man who jumped from behind a pyracantha bush in the park with his penis hanging out. I turned and ran all the way home.

There was a man who called me to clean his apartment. He locked me in and wouldn't let me out until I beat him off.

There was a man who knew my mother, said he'd give me a ride to my girlfriend's house, then stopped halfway there near an empty field. He forced himself on me, tried to have me in the awkwardness of the car seat. I cried and told him I was a virgin. He said if I gave him a hand job, he would let me go.

All the while I never talked about these times. There were too many for them not to be my fault, they had made me dirty, but I heard you tell me I was innocent—the young girls are innocent—and I believe you. I believe you and I will write.

PAT PARKER

"At nine years old, being a black child in the South in the 1950s, it was impossible for my story to have any other ending, and that still makes me angry."

Pat Parker was born on January 20, 1944, in Houston, Texas, where her story, "Shoes," takes place. About the story, she writes: "I felt the need to get it out of my system in order to move on to other things. I had never told the story to anyone. I carried a great deal of anger as a result of the incident: anger toward my parents for their insistence that I respect any adult as an authority figure; anger toward the store owner for his perversion and use of me; and anger at the economic structure of this political system."

She continues: "I still have thoughts from time to time of returning to Houston and seeing if that store is still there. I often wonder about the store owner and his family. And I wonder how many other little girls, long after I left the school, were invited in to see the shoes."

"Shoes" was originally published in True to Life Adventure Stories, *edited by Judy Grahn and published by Diana Press. Four books of poetry by Pat Parker have also been published, and she has appeared on three record albums and in numerous anthologies. She is the author of several books of poetry as well as a novel and a play. She is also a director of the Oakland Feminist Health Center in Oakland, California.*

* * *

Pat Parker's last book, Jonestown and Other Madness, *was published by Firebrand Books in 1985. In June 1989, she died of cancer after a lifetime of contribution to lesbian feminist literature, culture, and survival.*

Shoes

"Gal, don't you ever do that again. You hear me?"

"Yes, daddy."

Victor released his daughter's arm and laid down his belt. Frances ran off to her room. She could hear her father still raging to her mother.

"That girl's gonna cost me all my jobs. Mr. Clark said she was downright insolent to him on the phone. She's got to understand that white folks don't like being talked to like that. They decide that she's too uppity, and that reflects on me. They'll stop calling and then what'll we do?"

"Now, Victor, calm down. She's young. She don't understand yet about these things."

"Well, dammit! She better start! It don't hurt nobody to say yessir to nobody. That girl is just too smart for her own good. Hell, she talks to me sometimes like I'm a child. All those damn teachers and books are getting to her head."

Frances turned over in her bed. She was angry. She had not done anything wrong. She had answered the phone; told the man that her father wasn't home. She'd written down his name and number, said goodbye, and hung up. The only thing she hadn't done was punctuate her sentences with sirs. Why was it so important to say sir? That was for people you respected a great deal. She didn't even know the man on the phone. For all she knew, he could have been a drinker or gambler. Anything. She ran her fingers over her body. She could feel the sting from the belt and trace the outline of the welts beginning to form. But she didn't cry. No matter how long and hard he hit her, she wouldn't cry. And she knew that got to him. I can't stop him from whipping me, but I don't have to cry. And that gets him every time. She smiled at the thought.

Victoria cries if daddy looks at her funny. And Janice and Reba will cry if he whips them, but not me. She was tougher than any of her sisters and she was the youngest. I'll never let him see me cry.

She had come to know her father well in her ten years. In the summer, he would often take her to work with him. They moved from used-car dealer to used-car dealer. He would drag his six-foot frame from his car and put on his smile. "Howdy do, Mr. Whoever. Need any tires cut today?" And they would pause. "Well, Victor, lemme see. Yeah, I think we got a few over in the shed. Go on over and see Mr. Whoever." He would smile his grateful smile, take his stool and retreading iron, and go find Mr. Whoever. While he worked, she would amuse herself by climbing among the stacks of old tires. And when she tired of that, she would find an old magazine in one of the showrooms and sit and read. Some days there would be many tires and she would go get in her father's car and pretend she was some rich person, or an outlaw escaping from jail. Some days she would be a rich king, or a lonely rich boy with no parents. Or she'd be on a big ranch with as many horses as a person could have.

At least once a month, her father would decide that he'd earned enough money to take care of the family and they would go fishing. She loved to go fishing with her father. When she was eight, he had bought her her own rod and reel. Now instead of sitting with a line and old meat hoping to snare a crab, she got to sit on the banks with him and fish like the grown-ups. Sometimes they took the rest of the family. She didn't like those times. Her sisters and mother would complain all the time about going home. When she and her father went alone, they would stay all day and well into the night.

Those were the good times; but she also knew her father on the days when there were no tires to cut. Then the house was silent with the fear of his rage. The chickens and rabbits were inspected very carefully. If the animal's water seemed the least bit yellow, she would be whipped. Any little thing wrong and his belt would be off his waist, wrapped around his hands, and flying through the air at his target. She had seen him and felt him whip her and her sisters until her mother had grabbed him. Seen her mother stand painfully by and watch until he seemed out of control and then take him into the bedroom to find the man again. And she had learned not to cry. She was whipped more often and longer. His face would contort and his words would shatter sanity, but she would not cry. And her mother would stop him and she would lead him into their bedroom, his shoulders slumped and his step heavy. She would stand and watch, her eyes glaring, standing very tall. She would not cry, and she was the victor.

There was a new store. The vacant building behind the green pole that served as a signal for the Pioneer Bus Line to stop and pick up the black people and take them from one ward to another had been transformed into an ocean of shoes. Frances stood and peered in the window. The large cardboard figure of Buster Brown and Tyge smiled back at her and she thought of the commercial.

> My name's Buster Brown,
> I live in a shoe.
> This is my Dog Tyge—
> He lives in there too.

Red and Terry approached her. "Hey, Frances, let's play some peg."

"Naw, I don't want to."

Red and Terry were her friends. Each day after school, they would come to the bus stop and play games while waiting for the green bus to take them home. They couldn't play together in school. The boys and the girls were each sent to their respective parts of the playgrounds. Frances hated playing with the other girls. They didn't like to play football or baseball. They only wanted to play silly girl games and giggle. But after school, she could play what she wanted. If the ground was dry, they would produce little sacks of marbles, and fire missiles into a crude circle to destroy their opponents. If the ground was wet, they would produce rusty pocketknives and play peg. They were good friends. They always returned each other's marbles, and they never tried to break each other's knife in peg.

This day she didn't want to play. She watched the man in the store put one pair of shoes here, another there. She had never seen so many different kinds of shoes. Her entire world of shoes consisted of brown-and-white saddle oxfords for school, black patent leather for Sunday, and sneakers for play. Here in this store were red shoes, blue shoes, white shoes, sandals, boots, grown-up shoes, kid shoes, the high laced old-lady shoes, all kinds of shoes.

"Hey, Frances, here comes the bus."

All the way home, Frances thought about the shoes. She imagined herself rich and having all those shoes in her house. She watched herself changing shoes every hour and then throwing them away. She would never have to polish shoes again. She would never have to take off a pair of shoes before she could play. She could run in the mud or water and not worry about getting whipped. She wouldn't have to have taps to keep them from running over. She spent the rest of the day feeling good. Tomorrow she would get to see the shoes again.

Frances stayed after school that day and helped her teacher clean the boards and check the desks and cloakroom for forgotten articles. She knew that Red and Terry would be at the bus stop wondering where she was. But she didn't want to see them. They would want to play some game. She would take her time and let them go home. Then she could look at the shoes. They wouldn't understand if she told them about the fantasies. They would laugh. It would be better if she just let them go home.

When she reached the bus stop, they were gone. She walked to the window and looked in. She saw herself a great dancer on television wearing the blue ballet slippers. People stood up and applauded her performance, throwing roses on the stage. She took her bows and smiled.

"What are you doing?"

"Huh! Nothing . . . sir."

Frances looked up at the white man. She had almost forgotten, but the memory of her recent whipping swept across her mind. She had seen this man before. Yes, he was the man in the shoe shop. She smiled.

"What's your name, little girl?"

"Frances, sir."

"You live around here, Frances?"

"No, sir, I live in Sunnyside. I'm waiting for the bus."

"Sunnyside. That's a long way from here. You know how to go all that way by yourself?"

"Yessir. I do it every day. I'm a big girl now. I'm in the fifth grade."

"Would you like to come inside and look at the shoes, Frances?"

"Oh, yessir."

Frances couldn't believe what was happening. This had to be the nicest man in the world. She felt really important. It was almost like she was going to buy some shoes.

"It's almost time for me to go, so I'm going to close up the shutters, Frances. You go ahead and look around."

Frances walked slowly around the display tables. Barely touching first one shoe, then another. She would wear that shoe to the movie, and that shoe to the park, and that shoe to the rodeo, and that shoe to the circus, and—

"Would you like to go in the back and see where we store the shoes?"

"Yessir."

Frances followed the man into the little room. She stopped inside the door and he turned and beckoned her to a small stool. She sat and looked around the room. There were rows and rows of boxes. It was more fun to see the shoes in the other room. She wondered if the man would give her a pair of shoes. He closed the door and turned to her.

"Do you like candy, Frances?"

"Yessir."

At first she hadn't noticed the man walk up to her. He had unzipped his pants and was holding a large red thing, stroking it back and forth. His eyes were funny-looking, like he was nervous.

"Do you know what this is?"

"No, sir."

"Well, this is like candy, and I want you to suck it. And when you're finished, I'll give you a present."

Frances looked at the large red thing. It didn't look very much like any candy she had seen. It looked like a long, large, red mushroom. There was something white in the middle coming out of a hole. She looked at the man.

"Go on, Frances, suck it."

He tilted her head and pushed the large red thing into her mouth. It felt hard and much too big. And it didn't taste sweet at all like candy. The man had his hand around Frances's neck. His grip tightened.

"Suck it, up and down, like candy."

Frances was frightened. She didn't know what to do. She didn't like this candy. She didn't like the way the man sounded. His voice was mean like her father's. She felt like she was going to throw up, and she was afraid she'd be beaten. All of a sudden the man let out a cry. He pulled away from her and she stared as white cream came spurting from the large red thing, which was becoming smaller. She didn't know what to do. She knocked over the stool and backed away from the man. He had taken a handkerchief from somewhere and was wiping the red thing. He pushed it back into his pants.

"Now, didn't you like that, Frances?"

"Yessir."

"Tomorrow, after school, you come back and we'll do it again. But you mustn't tell anyone about it. It's our little game. Okay?"

"Yessir."

The man led Frances to the door. He reached into his pocket and handed her a quarter. He unlocked the front door and let her out.

"Now remember. It's our private game."

Frances didn't answer. She saw the green bus and ran to it. She didn't like the game. She looked at the quarter clutched in her hand. She dropped it on the floor of the bus.

She was very quiet that evening at home. Her mother checked her forehead to see if she had a fever. She went to bed that night and she did not think about the shoes.

The next afternoon after school, Frances talked Red and Terry into catching the bus at the next bus stop. She told them the man in the shoe store would probably take their knives if they played peg in front of his store. They never played there again.

MARTHA ROGERS

"My mother remembered this story in enough detail to tell me about it some fifty years after it happened."

In "A Street Fair," Martha Rogers (a pseudonym) describes a molestation experience that happened to her mother. Martha wrote the story for her mother, who is now over seventy years old. She did not tell Martha about this incident until four years earlier. "I am sure she never discussed it with her own mother," Martha writes. "My grandmother was a strict and puritanical woman."

When she told the story to Martha, she did it in a matter-of-fact way. "Yet she did say she could remember feeling sick and dirty and ashamed at the time it happened," Martha continues. Martha's mother taught school for many years and is now retired and living in Arizona with her husband of forty years.

A Street Fair

I had brushed my hair till it sparkled, golden, and ma tied in a blue gingham bow to match my sundress. Jack's taking me to the fair. Pa took the others already, but Jack's taking me. He's my best brother. He never pushes me or calls me names. He's big and strong and calls me a peasquatch. He's twelve.

"Wow, what a pretty-looking peasquatch!"

Jack takes my hand and we walk to the fair. It's right in the
middle of town. They've blocked off Main Street and set a Ferris
wheel smack in front of Jones Drug Store. I can see it turning
people high in the air, then down again, round and round. It's
noisy with music and screaming and laughing.

"Jack, look, candy apples."

"You don't waste any time, do you, Celey. Okay, we'll get
one."

Jack gets a candy apple for me and one for him. They are big
and shiny red. I lick mine and Jack takes a mouthful of his. Our
lips are red as we smile at each other.

"Hey, look, Celey."

I look, see nothing but legs walking, bumping through the
street. The whole town must be here!

"I can't see, Jack. What? What?"

"Come on, let's go closer. It's snakes. Want to see some snakes,
Celey?"

Jack grabs my hand and pulls me through the crowd. We stop
at a wooden circle fence someone has put up right in the street.
Lots of people are pressed close to the fence, looking. I hang my
elbows over the edge and boost myself up on my toes so I can see,
too.

A dark man without a shirt stands in the middle of the circle,
snakes winding in and out around him like hair braiding, unbraid-
ing. He holds a black snake taller than me. It thrusts its tongue at
him and they stare at each other. Once I caught a snake down by
the pond, but he was small, more like a worm. I remember his
eyes, though, round beady little eyes, and he'd looked happy
somehow. These snakes exploring the street inside the fence have
the same smiling look, but they throb with excitement or fear as
the man stands among them and the people press close.

It is hard to breathe. The air is thick with snake smells; musty,
sweaty-sweet, grown-up. Most of the snakes are plain brown or

black, but one is the color of my ma's hair, brown and golden. One has orange faces on his back like a jack-o'-lantern. He winds his body around a long brown snake and the two of them curl under and over, rolling in a snake dance.

The snakes' skins glisten in the sunlight. One little green snake slithers quickly over a pile of bigger snakes. He comes over right below me where I am peeking over the fence and looks up at me. He wants out, I can feel it. Poor little green snake. We are friends; we have passed a look.

People talk louder now, moving in their places, watching the man in the ring. I look, too. The snake winds around the man's arms, across his neck. Like my green friend, the black snake watches me, showing off his white markings. Why doesn't the snake bite the man? I'll ask Jack. He knows almost everything.

A hand pats me. Jack? I turn my face up to a man's face. He smiles. He has only a few teeth and his smell is rotten apples. I move over, around the fence. Where is Jack?

Standing taller on my toes, I search the faces along the fence for my brother's face. All the eyes watch the snakes, all the mouths talk and laugh, making too much noise.

Rubbing. The man is close again. Behind me, rubbing my bottom. I want my brother. I don't like this smiling man. Again I push my way around the fence.

The snakes hiss and thrust their tongues.

Now I smell the rotten-apple man behind me, his face near my shoulder, resting on my hair. He is so close. And his hand is on me, rubbing me, his finger probing, darting, like the snakes, around and around. I'm going to throw up.

There is Jack across the ring.

"Jack, Jack!"

The man moves away. Jack comes to me, taking my hand. He's with a friend from school.

"Do you like the snakes, Celey?"

"Jack, I don't feel good."

"Too much candy apple, huh. Me 'n' Kevin will take you home. Come on."

Jack and Kevin make a queen's chair with their arms and carry me through the crowd to our house.

"Oh, hurry, Jack, I'm so sick."

Jack calls to ma, "Too much fair for Celey."

Ma looks at me, smiles. "Go on up and lie down, honey. I'll be up in a minute. Thanks, Jack and Kevin. Was it the candy apples? She never knows when to stop eating those candy apples."

Up the stairs to the bathroom; I vomit, heaving, crying. Don't hear me, ma, don't hear me. I cry and vomit some more. Finally it's over and I run water in the bathtub, get in, and scrub hard all over. Ma comes then, helps me dry off and get into my nightgown.

"I'll bring some tea. You'll feel better—just rest for a while."

And summer goes and comes and goes and comes again until now I am grown. Eighteen years old. So many years have passed, I'd forgotten the snakes and the man and the smell. Until tonight.

Now I am a wife. Today I wore a white gown. It was a fine wedding, the finest in the county, they all said. I never looked at another boy but you, never kissed, no one has pressed my body. I've saved myself, just like ma taught me. You are good and kind. I love you, I do.

But as you sleep beside me, naked, the musty man-smell of your body mixes with the rotten apple of too much champagne and no matter how I bite my hand to forget, I think of the snakes, the throbbing snakes, the man touching.

KATE MILLETT

"This episode, which indeed was something I never told anyone, had to be expressed before anything else in my autobiography could take form."

Kate Millett, born on Sept. 14, 1934, in St. Paul, Minnesota, is often regarded as one of the pioneering theoreticians of the women's liberation movement. In Sexual Politics, *published in 1970, she attacked the patriarchal nature of society as the root cause of feminine oppression. She is also the author of* The Prostitution Papers *(1973),* Flying, *her autobiography, and* Sita *(1977).*

About the piece we have excerpted from Flying, *she writes: "This was the first section of* Flying, *which was composed, written in fact before I had any idea of what the book would become. I wondered at it at the time, knew inside that it was the most secret, desperate information I should have to divulge—and then wondered more: what could I even do with these paragraphs, make of them? I even took refuge in persuading myself that they were an exercise in style, the influence of Faulkner ('time is so long,' etc.). Nonsense. They were the germ of the book, the germ of autobiography itself, the transcendence of shame."*

* * *

Kate Millett's most recent book is The Loony-Bin Trip, *published in 1990 by Simon & Schuster.*

215

from Flying

Something remembered from childhood. Waiting for the bus in a
snowstorm. Corner of Cleveland and Highland Park Road. Highland Drug behind me in the wind. Warm in there. And they got
chocolate malts. But if the bus doesn't see anyone, it goes right
on. Better wait outside. Ain't got the extra quarter anyway. Can
still see the black iron fence of the convent. Slowly disappearing
in the snow. We have such a big campus 'cause Derham is the
prep school for St. Kate's. I hold all my books in front of me,
proud there are so many. This week is the first big tests. French
today. Wonder how I did. History tomorrow. The cold is like
being sick. The sulfa drugs when I had mastoid. Dr. Flannigan
said I was delirious. Wonderful word. Blue car stops for the light.
Mercury. Hard to see. Going to be a real blizzard. He's opening
the door. Gonna give me a ride. Must be one of Daddy's drafts-
men. Why else would he stop? Inside I see his face. But it's not
Swanny or one of the other ones. Don't know all of them too well.
Their faces come and go, back door to the basement. When I go
down to check my math on Daddy's machine, they tease me.
Look again. Sort of red hair. Nothing familiar. I must convert it to
a known face while he is busily fussing over the door. Making
sure I don't fall out. So considerate. Locking it. He says stuff
about the weather, how cold I must be. Don't know what to say,
but I must be polite. Thank him lots of times. Shall we take the
river road? The houses of the rich, the trees, the Mississippi.
Sure. My favorite way. Of course he knows where I live, friend of
the family I am just too dumb to recognize. Mother says I don't
pay attention. We turn down toward the river, history test, comfort of warmth, security, convenience. Sense of protection so familiar. I am a girl. People take care of me. The man is talking.
Now it seems he needs to remember where I live. Across from St.
Thomas College. People think that means Summit Avenue. But

it only means Selby. I should remember to say *back* of St. Thomas. There is something funny that he doesn't know where I live. Maybe everything's wrong. Never mind the voice in my stomach saying he's a stranger. Little rise of fear in my gut. He pressed the button on my side. Locked in. Warnings about men in cars. He mustn't know I am thinking this. Guy's being nice. Saw I was a kid waiting for the bus, dark coming on, going to be terrible tonight. Sure, he's being nice. Giving me a ride home. I am wearing my uniform. Doesn't make sense, thinking these things about him. He's asking about my briefcase. I am holding it in front of me, brand-new today. Real or imitation? New, my first briefcase. Real, but imitation leather. I admit it. He grabs toward it laughing but touches my front. Breasts, mother says. Sally my big sister says bosoms. So embarrassing. This is a mistake. His laugh is scary—my face is hot. It is not happening. No, the car is not going to stop here with only trees around us. No. There are no houses in this part of the river road. Gray darkness quiet. I refuse this. Deny too that I see his big hands shoving themselves into my blouse. Regulation with a V neck and three cuff buttons. So it can't be. Just not possible the red hands fumbling below my skirt. Trying to enter its Derham Hall accordion pleats. The black serge makes this crazy. Great purple flesh in his lap long huge horrible. Is that what one looks like? This is real now. It's danger. Wild dream awake in the gray evening. Here is the expected terror at last. We are partners. We do things by signals. I am yelling the Virgin Mary, my school, the sin against chastity. But it sounds silly. Every day we say the Blessed Virgin—but we don't scream it. I'm shouting. But there is sometimes no sound because my throat is closed. He will not be able to put the purple thing inside me. That must be what he wants, grabbing to touch me we fight over my underpants his finger hurting me. The purple thing would not fit. He will not be able to do it. He is there and I am here. He must stop the car first 'cause we are still moving. If I could get out. Run away but he's so ₐᵤch bigger. Stronger, hurting me. Now we are wrestling over the door and the button on the door. Is he hitting me? Calling me names. Little bitch. Slut. I run. How can I run if my legs don't work. Run and fall in the snow. Throwing up. Crawl. Hide in the trees. He circles the empty lot in his car. The blue Mercury slowly going around the space where I am, the place without a road where I hide watching it. Time is so long. When he is at the other end, I can break and cross. Up the hill. Running with the air blue in the snow. Watching the car disappear is mercy. Then go for the hill. Running the six miles home and halfway there at St. Clair—I discover I have lost it. My turtle. The brace to keep my teeth straight. Spit it out in the snow. I have lost twenty-five dollars. Again. And the last time I promised them. Mother said they could never afford to buy another. Pink plastic in the new white powder almost dark outside the car among the trees. Snow six inches deep. Dark now. I cannot go back and find it. At dinner a fever till they find out it is lost. It is my fault. They must never know how.

Telling on him is telling on me. The pneumonia is weakness, skin hot all the time, dizzy when you sit up. Both lungs. It sounded so important. In the hospital I was special. Got presents. People came to see me. Even Nancy came. The nurse kids me about the shots. "Turn over for another one in your pincushion," she says. But at home now it is just boring. Lunchtime Mrs. Luger comes to make me a sandwich. Campbell's tomato soup. Mother goes out to work. Daddy is gone now. Now I don't have a father. At school I lie and say he's just out of town. In Greenland building an air base. It's only partly true. Of course he's up there in the ice, he sent us a card, but he's never coming back. Mother found out about him. Told me when I drove her up Cathedral Hill, so icy if I don't pay attention we'll roll backwards the way I do when Sally teaches me and she yells. Thirteen. Can't pass the test for two more years. "Looks like Daddy's car," I said. Black Merc bigger than Mother's little Ford. Harder to drive, you can't see the edges of it. "Yes," she says, "it's your father's car." Now I see there's a lady driving it. Can't be his. She still says it is. "It's time you knew your father has a mistress." Word out of a book. Hearing her and still driving while she says Daddy is going to leave, she can't stand it anymore, voice gagging as it has for years at the dinner table, chokes on her food. I drive along Summit past the Walker Houses like castles, my aunt on Daddy's side was married to Chip Walker. Asking, my hands terrified on the wheel, will I still get to see Aunt Christina now. Her house beckoning me like a lover down Virginia Avenue as we pass the corner. Why can't I be her daughter, live with her, no husband now, no kids of her own, all that money—I could even give some of it to Mother. Now we won't have any money. How will we live? My mind getting there before she even says it. And we must go home. We don't live up here. No, out in Midway near the river. Back of St. Thomas, and the trees stretch bare gray evening before dinner nights he doesn't come home. Now we won't have to wait dinner for him. Throws his hat in the door first. "You're drunk," her voice messy, then she cries and we hate the way she cries. Like an animal. Now it is just Mother and my little sister Mary. Sally went away to college. Escaped. Mother has a job but she can't make any money. And I'm sick. If I have to drop out of Derham 'cause it costs money I can't ever see Nancy again. She's my best friend.

Lying in bed sick I think about the man. The blue car. I touch myself and my head gets hot. It's a sin. A sin to have gotten in his car. I have been touched by him. Did I lose my virginity? What does it mean really? Not a sin if I escaped. Even if I ran away, was it a sin? But a sin to lose the turtle. Sometimes I want him back. He could put the thing in me. Then I would know what it is. If he put it in me I would stop itching. Look at the roses on the wallpaper, the yellow spot where Mary threw up once. Don't sin. Don't think about anything. Think about the basketball games at St. Thomas. Be one tonight, it's Friday, but I'm sick. The boys'll be there. Nancy'll be there too. Ashamed again, thinking that.

'Cause people act funny about us when we say we're in love. Before Thanksgiving vacation we told the seniors and they laughed, kind of scary, like when you've made a mistake. The nun heard and she got mad. Sally's boyfriend heard us talking on the phone and said a magic word to Mother. Lesbian. It takes so long to get well. Already it's eight weeks. Dr. Flannigan says six more. There's nothing to do but remember. Over and over. This secret. The blue Mercury. His face sort of blurry. The terrible purple thing. Then running. It keeps happening. If I yell no one hears me, the house is empty. Will he find out where I live, get me, tell on me? Face hot, sweating, is it the fever, I wonder. It's a sin and thinking is a sin. How do I stop it from happening?

ANN SIMONTON

"I used to think my personal power was contingent on my being a good sex object, something good to look at like cherry à la mode."

Ann Simonton was born in 1952 in Harlan County, Kentucky. When she was fourteen years old, she was enrolled in a modeling school. "Trophy Girl" is about her first public appearance as a model and the sexual abuse she had to tolerate. "Being a trophy girl was one of many public humiliations I came to endure professionally," Ann writes. "This instance was not the first or last time I was sexually abused by men. This piece symbolizes the ease with which I internalized male aggression. It was my place as a sex object to accept every insult or grab. Even my experience with rape I learned to swallow like toast in the morning."

Ann worked as a professional model for eleven years: "I often felt like a prostitute. Modeling was merely a socially acceptable form of using my sexuality to make money. I greatly resented the competition I was forced to engage in with other women. Our whole system is designed to cultivate this competition between women for male attention. This competitive block isolates us and perpetuates the status quo."

Ann has completed a book on her experiences as a fashion model and her transition to feminism. "Trophy Girl" is an excerpt from that book. She is also an activist committed to improving women's image in the media. "I'd go to any length," she states, "to provide healthy alternatives to the stereotype of women as helpless Barbie dolls."

Trophy Girl

"Oh, mama, what am I supposed to wear?" I wailed, rummaging through my drawers of clothes. "I don't own one decent bathing suit!"

"Ask Meg for her orange and white striped one, honey," mama called from the next room.

I was so jittery. I had never been a Trophy Girl before or made a public appearance anything like this one. This was my first official modeling job and I was filled with terror.

I knew the duties of a Trophy Girl from old Steve McQueen movies. She had to give the winner of the car race a trophy and a kiss. The very thought of having to do that, within a matter of hours, hounded me as I dashed around the house looking for nylons and Meg's suit. When I found the swimsuit, I tried it on for mama.

"Looks great," she assured me.

"It does?" I asked doubtfully. The suit was equipped with hard-cupped bosoms that were crunchy and brittle with age. The whole top half of the suit stood out on its own, barely touching my undeveloped, fourteen-year-old chest. I felt ridiculous, pretending to be something I wasn't. But as I scrutinized myself in mama's vanity mirror, I decided she knew best.

While under the shower, I carefully shaved the four or five hairs that had just begun to show in my armpits. After removing some bristle from my legs and thighs, I scrubbed my scalp clean. After drying off, I began the tedious battle with my hair. I hated it for being brown and curly when the style was blond and straight. My hair was still growing out from a horrible Beatle cut I had gotten a year before. I rolled it on oversize curlers anyway and sat under the hair dryer praying for a perfect flip.

As the hot air began to steam my head, I worried about being too inexperienced for the job. Maybe I hadn't taken enough modeling classes. I wished now I hadn't been so eager to accept the offer. I'd taken it because I knew mama would want me to. Besides, why else was I going to modeling school? You were supposed to take every job offered, as part of the learning process. So I kept silent.

I couldn't even eat one of my favorite meals, fish fried with cornmeal, lima beans, and green salad that mama had made. Instead I gulped some iced tea and resumed the struggle with my hair and face. I stretched a smudgy line of black eyeliner across my lids. Blinking too soon left huge wet marks near both eyebrows. Wiping them off, I smeared more white shadow at the arch of my brow and flicked my lashes with a gooey wand of brown mascara.

"Doesn't anybody have some nude pantyhose I could borrow?" I yelled. No answer. "What shoes, mama? I can't wear flats, can I?" I was desperate. It was almost time to leave.

Daddy was already out warming up the car. Mama brought down her black heels. "You don't need nylons, honey," she said. "Let's go."

I flinched at the sight of her shoes. My God, high heels. I'd never survive the night. Slipping her shoes on, I went to the mirror for a final check. My image reassured me; I was no prize, but close enough. My two sisters, Meg and Catey, filed out to the car with mama. It was Friday night; my older sisters, Susan and Mary, had dates and couldn't come. I threw an old sweater over my shoulders and came flying out. I was relieved that my family was going with me. They made me feel safe and proud.

On the ride to the racetrack, we discussed mainly how to get there, since we *never* went to such events. My insides knotted tight as we approached the speedway; anxiety always hit me in the gut. But I was determined to fool everyone, including myself, by acting like an experienced model. The die was cast; there was no turning back now.

At the gate I explained I was the Trophy Girl. They ushered

me to one side as my family purchased their tickets. A large man wearing a cowboy hat and excessive turquoise jewelry handed me a banner and pointed his finger. "Go right over to section A, doll," he said. "That's where you're gonna stand."

Breathing deeply, I shrank into a corner until mama came through the gate. She helped me drape the identity sash across my chest. It read: PAT QUINLAN MODELS. We couldn't get it to hang right. The whole getup embarrassed me. I thought I would die if anyone I knew recognized me—and at a racetrack, of all places. Finally mama gave up on the sash, assuring me, "You look fine, sweetie. Give me your sweater and go on."

Reluctantly stripping off my covering, I walked the long distance to section A with unsteady steps. I had never cared for car racing, finding the noise and smells offensive. The sport itself seemed stupid—men jumping into souped-up cars labeled with the names of motor-oil or auto-accessory sponsors, then blasting around the track hoping to win a trophy and a kiss. What strange entertainment!

I stood there looking at the ground, wishing I could fade into the background. I wanted to shield my nakedness from the crowd's gawking eyes. But modeling was what I had so *wanted* to do. Wasn't this a pinnacle of sorts? Why wasn't I having fun?

The hot rods went spinning by me, screeching as they cornered the oblong field. I choked on the stench of burning rubber and black oily fumes that filled my lungs. Standing close to the track, I tried to casually plug my ears as the cars thundered by.

Finally when the first race was over, a man identified by the loudspeaker as Clem Dickson climbed out of his machine. The winner? My heart sank. He was fat and old, maybe thirty years my senior. There had to be some mistake. It wasn't supposed to happen this way. Winners were blond young men with broad, handsome grins. But then again, I wasn't blond myself, so what could I expect?

My body stiffened as Dickson started toward me. Fighting an

urge to run, I forced a weak smile and handed him the trophy. Grinning back, he drawled, "'Preciate it, ma'am." Coming toward me, his arms outstretched, he clutched me roughly and darted his soppy tongue into my mouth. As I struggled backward, his wet sausage hands grasped me even tighter. I panicked, afraid he would never let go. The crowd began cheering and whistling wildly. I realized I couldn't make a scene. My job compelled me to endure this sweaty, liquor-breathing stranger.

I was finally able to break away from his grip and I ran back to the grandstand where my family sat watching. I looked up at them, trying to smile. Mama's knowing, sympathetic look seemed to acknowledge that my experience had been anguishing.

I felt ashamed. My chin sank to my chest. I couldn't bear to look at the crowd. I felt as if, somehow, it had been my fault that such an ugly man had won. Possibly if I had been better-looking, he would have been better-looking, too. Boys never noticed me at school, a sure sign that I wasn't pretty. My body was wrong, my pale skin was freckled and pimpled, my suit was old-fashioned, and even the crooked sash proclaimed my imperfection.

I tried my best to walk like a model back to my station to watch the next heat. One more trophy and I could go home. The black-and-white checkered flags flew in the air as the fans began to yell. The spectators didn't seem to notice the Trophy Girl's inadequacy.

Trying to maintain a cheerful look, I endured the final explosion of racing motors and screaming fans until the second race was over. The winner was—my luck!—Clem Dickson again. He lumbered to the winner's circle to receive his second trophy of the night.

This time I was steeled for his advances. I made our kiss short and abrupt. Chagrined, he realized he wasn't going to get any more out of me. As I stepped back, a balding flagman grabbed me from behind and turned me around for his kiss. What had I done to warrant this? Had I smiled in his direction? I blamed his lust on my presence and let him get away with it.

The newspaper photographer approached and snapped a shot of Dickson and me. Afterward, the photographer sidled up to me insisting that I call him later that night, or *any time*. I was learning quickly what to expect as a model. Was this what I was paying a lot of money for—to learn how to attract this kind of attention? Even so, the school had failed to tell me how to handle it once I got it. Was I obligated to accept grabs, kisses, stares, and whistles, and keep right on smiling?

The ride home with my family was long and quiet. I decided that if the experience were really as bad as it seemed, mama would say something or forbid me to take any more modeling jobs like that. Since she didn't, the disgust I felt must be a childish reaction. I felt very alone.

It was after ten o'clock by the time we got home so we all went straight to bed. I slowly climbed the stairs up to the room Catey and I shared and sluggishly peeled off Meg's suit. Catey was already in our bed, flopping around.

"Hurry up, Annie, it's chilly in here!" she said.

I slipped my nightgown over my head and climbed in quietly beside her. Sensing my mood, Catey asked, "Is something the matter?"

"I dunno." I turned away from her.

"That guy was creepy, huh?"

I turned to look straight in her eyes. "Yeah, Catey, he was *really* creepy."

"It was awful, huh?"

"Yeah, it was." I turned off the light.

"Let's snuggle up tonight, okay?" she suggested.

"Sure, Cate." With both our heads toward the balcony doors, we wrapped our bodies close for warmth.

"G'night, Ann," Catey mumbled sleepily.

I held her tightly and fought back the tears blurring my eyes.

"G'night, Cate. Sweet dreams."

MAUREEN BRADY

"I've never thought of dealing with the molestation as separate from dealing with living within patriarchy."

Maureen Brady was born in New York in 1943 and soon there-after moved to Florida, where the molestation described in "Chiggers" occurred. Out of a confused sense of shame, she did not tell anyone about the incident. "This was an early experience in feeling 'adult,'" she writes, "not only because of the sexual feelings but because of the isolation of keeping something to one-self. I also think my sense of shame was connected not to how I felt intrinsically but to the extrinsic framework that meant telling others would bring in the component of shame.

"How I heal myself," she continues, "is to try to find construc-tive channels for anger. I find them in writing and in political organizing. I am also healed by being nurtured by the love of women."

"Chiggers" was originally published in Feminary. *Maureen's first novel,* Give Me Your Good Ear, *was published by Spinsters, Ink, which she cofounded, and in England by the Women's Press Ltd. Her second novel,* Folly, *was published by the Crossing Press Feminist Series in 1982.*

* * *

Maureen Brady's most recent book is The Question She Put to Herself, *published in 1987 by Crossing Press.*

227

Chiggers

Alone in the tree hut, Ginny stretched out her full length on the couch she and Zeke and Jack had worked on the week before. It was made from a couple of planks nailed to two-by-fours and covered with armfuls of pine needles and Spanish moss. She relaxed. The only concern that intruded on her comfort was the idea that there might be chiggers in the Spanish moss, but they had been sitting on the couch for almost a week now, and no one had turned up with any bites yet. She had heard of chiggers having an incubation time while they crawl around under the skin, inside the person, before they start biting to get back out. Probably that was something her mother had said, but she wasn't sure, and she couldn't remember how long they took, either. Her mother said lots of things about the woods that she didn't listen to very well because she liked playing in the woods—exploring, finding tracks, building the tree hut, listening to the noises—and most of the things her mother said were meant to make you not like the woods so well. Her mother was a lover of civilization.

She heard twigs crack in the clearing behind the tree hut, but she didn't bother getting up to use the lookout hole since she figured it would be her brother. Their house was just through the woods on the other side of the clearing. Zeke's house was in the opposite direction. They had chosen their tree deliberately to be halfway between the two subdivisions they lived in.

Jack climbed the ladder, which was made of boards nailed to the tree, and stuck his head into the hut. Because of the way the tree branched into two main trunks, the entrance to the hut was almost in the middle of the floor. "Where's Zeke?" he asked.

"How would I know?"

"He said he was coming."

"He probably had to change the baby's diaper."

Jack hiked himself the rest of the way into the hut and sat with his back against the opposite wall from Ginny. "Probably," he agreed. "I sure am glad Marty's getting potty-trained."

"Me, too," Ginny said.

"I hope mom doesn't have any more babies."

"She won't. She's too old. I heard her say so."

"Good," Jack said, leaving it at that, although he didn't understand what Ginny meant.

Ginny was in seventh grade, Jack was in fifth. "You'll get it in sixth grade," she said.

When Zeke came in, he sat up against the wall next to Jack even though Ginny got up to make more room on the couch. "I saw Shirley on the bus," Zeke said. "She's coming over as soon as she can."

"Shall we light up?" Ginny asked.

"Let's wait for Shirley," Jack said.

Shirley was Jack's girlfriend. She didn't come every day like the three of them because she had to baby-sit her kid sister most of the time, but when she did come, they played kissing games. Now there was an edge of anticipation in all of them that they didn't have when they were busy with planning, designing, hammering on, and surveying their work with the hut.

"Go ahead and roll it anyway, Zeke," Ginny said.

Zeke opened the tin box and took out the cigarette papers and the tobacco. They took turns stealing from their parents, and Zeke's dad rolled his own, so they had to settle for this when it was his turn. Ginny watched Zeke's hands as he performed the ritual. He brought the cigarette to his mouth and licked the glue on the paper. He had a small, slippery tongue. When they kissed, the tip of it sometimes came through to Ginny's lips by mistake. Zeke's eyes were dark and shiny and looked up at Ginny, smiling. He tapped the cigarette on the tin box, packing it. His hands were soft and small, smaller than Ginny's.

When Shirley arrived, they smoked the cigarette. Ginny paid attention to the fact that Shirley was a good smoker, she didn't just blow the smoke out in mouthfuls. Ginny wasn't sure why Shirley would want to take up with her brother, who turned green and got sick half the time when they smoked. Of course he didn't ever puke in front of Shirley, but would wait until he and Ginny were walking home and then puke in front of her. And just after Shirley had been kissing him, Ginny couldn't help but think.

Zeke ground out the cigarette butt with the heel of his sneaker. There was an awkward moment when they reshuffled so that Zeke and Ginny were together on the couch and Shirley and Jack were huddled in the corner.

"We gotta build another couch," Jack said.

"Yeah, tomorrow," Zeke said. "Tomorrow morning we're going to work on that hole in the roof; then we'll build another couch." While he said this, he took Ginny's hand and squeezed it tightly with his. Ginny looked over and saw that Jack was holding Shirley's hand even though he was talking to and looking at Zeke.

"For today we'll trade off," Jack said.

"Yeah," Zeke said.

Finally, he looked at Ginny. He seemed like a complete stranger to her, which was ridiculous since he was not only her boyfriend but also Jack's best friend and because their heads were so close she could smell his hair tonic, which had a putrid odor to it. They stared into each other's eyes, watching for some signal that would indicate it was time to advance their mouths across the gap between them. Ginny resisted the temptation to look across at Jack and Shirley to see if they had started yet. Then Zeke's lips reached Ginny's and they both closed their eyes at once and concentrated on coordinating the kiss. Zeke's lips were thicker than Ginny's and tended to cover her mouth completely so that she had to worry about keeping her nose from being blocked off by his cheek in order to be able to breathe. They held this lip-pressing kiss for a very long time with occasional variations, some intentional, some not—a squeeze of the hand, a slip of the tongue, a cold, bare tooth mistakenly taking part. Ginny was careful about keeping the rest of their body parts from touching by making sure she stretched her neck instead of sitting closer, and Zeke was careful about where he put his other hand. Usually he held it on the back of Ginny's neck, and sometimes, while he worked his lips into undulations that made her think of earthworms, he squeezed the back of her neck and sent chills up and down her spine.

Soon after they started kissing, Ginny always wondered about how they were going to reach an agreement in silence to all stop at once. Somehow they always did. Then they had a ritual of looking starry-eyed up through the hole in the roof to the sky and all saying, "Oh, boy. Oh, boy." This in spite of the fact that Ginny was always more excited by the prospect of the next session than by anything that had just transpired.

"Y'all come to my house in the morning," Zeke said, "so we can carry the boards over together. Wait'll you see what I got." Zeke lived in a newer subdivision than theirs, where lots of new houses were still being built, and so was their chief scavenger.

"See ya," Ginny said.

"See ya," Zeke responded, flashing his small hand up in a wave but keeping his eyes on Jack.

Ginny couldn't go with Jack to get the boards at Zeke's place the next morning because she had to stay with her sister while her mother went grocery shopping. She implored her mother to hurry home so that she might get into the woods in time to be part of the construction. Her mother gave her the same look that they all gave Marty whenever she stood in the middle of the room in her training pants and let the piddle run down her legs. Ginny turned her back on her mother's lack of approval and begged once more for her to hurry while her mother went on searching for the car keys.

As soon as the groceries were in the house, she took off. The

sun was strong. It was about eleven o'clock. She figured Zeke and
Jack would still be working on the roof, and they were. She could
hear the tap of the hammers as she started to cross the clearing.
About the same time she heard them, she saw the man. He was
sitting on the ground at the bottom of a tree at the far side of the
clearing. Twenty feet beyond that tree was their tree. Her first
thought was that he might own the land. On the west coast of
Florida in 1955, no one seemed to know who owned the spaces
that hadn't yet been chopped up into lots. She and Zeke and Jack
had made constant speculations about the landowner who would
probably come in and tear out the whole woods right from under
their tree hut and build a new subdivision. She had conjured up a
picture of him as a man with big feet who wore the hat of a
Texan despite the fact he was in Florida. This man under the tree
didn't fit the description, but still frightened Ginny and must
have sensed it.

"Don't be afraid," he said. "I'm just admiring your tree hut.
Did you make it?"

"Yes," she said. "Me and the boys."

Ginny felt self-conscious with him looking at her, but she felt it
would be impolite to just walk on by him. He was strange. She
had rarely seen an adult with nothing to do. She had seen old men
on porches, rocking away their time, but he wasn't that old. Still,
he was old to her, older than her father. He had a sad look to his
face, mushy soft and sad. His hair was gray and he had on a plaid
flannel shirt and tan work pants. Ginny was trying to figure out a
way to ask him if he owned the land when he said, "Here, sit
down here," indicating a place beside himself on the Spanish
moss. Ginny sat down like he said and worried again about the
chiggers. The man leaned back on his elbows, looked up at the
sky, and started making up things about the shapes of the clouds,
the way you can do with frost on a windowpane or with the face
of the moon. "Do you see that face?" he asked, pointing. "It's the
profile. See the nose, the lips? Very strong." His voice had a nice,

deep, rich sound to it, a little like her father's when he told sea stories.

She was wearing her white short shorts and her legs felt the heat of the sun. He moved a little closer while she was looking at the cloud that he said looked like a princess in a long white flowing gown. He said there were very few princesses in the real world. "But you might be one of them." Then she felt his hand very softly on her leg, and he started moving one finger back and forth a bit. It was so gentle she almost couldn't feel it, but she knew it was there. She could see it. Her throat dried up and she couldn't think of a way to tell him to move it. Her legs felt hot, as if they were blushing. He kept on looking up at the sky and making up more things about the clouds, and she had to keep looking up to pay attention. She couldn't really listen, though. She just couldn't move. She thought maybe Zeke or Jack would come down soon or call her, and then she would jump up and run. *But if one of them saw, she would die.*

He moved over even more, and she couldn't look down at his hand, but that one finger just kept moving back and forth, back and forth; she almost couldn't feel it, but it was closer to her privates, over by the inside of her leg. She didn't know why she couldn't think of anything to say. He seemed so sad. She knew she shouldn't just stay there and let him do that—the finger was moving up and down along the edge of her underpants then, right where her short shorts ended. He was talking all the time in his low, soft voice, and he was gentle. "You're an awfully sweet girl," he said. "I think you like clouds, too. You see those things I show you in them." She could feel his eyes on her cheek as if they were burning two nickel imprints into it. "Your parents are very lucky to have such a nice girl." She thought she ought to tell him they had two girls and a boy, but she couldn't talk, her mouth was too dry. She guessed that he didn't have a daughter. She didn't dare move. He seemed very connected to her, and she was afraid he might cry.

She prayed he would stop if she just stayed still. She didn't move a muscle, and it seemed as if she weren't even breathing. She kept thinking he had stopped, because she hadn't felt anything, but he hadn't. His touch was just so light, and she was almost numb.

He snuck the finger under the elastic of her underpants. She tried to pretend that she had imagined it, but then he started back and forth again.

"I have to go home for lunch now," she blurted.

"Oh, not so soon. You could wait just a little while, couldn't you?"

Of course she could. How could she lie to him? She was thinking she could say she heard her mother call, but he would've heard her, too. She thought it was his second finger. It was just making a light tickle, nothing to be scared of. He wasn't doing any real harm.

"Where did you get such nice hair?" he asked. "You know, you're a pretty girl."

She squirmed slightly, turning toward the clearing. It felt like an abrupt move and his eyes looked hurt, but she really had only moved an inch or two. His hand had followed her, never losing contact, as though it had become one of her own parts. He wasn't doing anything different, just the same back and forth, but she couldn't stand it. She did appreciate that he thought she was pretty, so she waited another minute, not to insult him. Then she jumped. On her feet in one motion. "Gotta go for lunch."

His eyes were fastened on her. "I'm a little hungry, too. Maybe you can bring me something back." He wasn't insulted or excited or anything, but his eyes were still burning through her. His stare reminded her of how she might look when she wanted a wish to come true, when she would stare intently across a room or up at the sky and ask God or her mother, "Please, please, grant me this."

"Okay," she said, and ran across the clearing toward the road, her heart making a tripping thump in her chest. Even when he was out of sight and she slowed down to a walk, her heart went on scaring her. She was headed for home, but she realized she couldn't go there yet without her mother wanting to know why she was back so soon. And how could she tell her? How could she explain that she hadn't been able to move? How could she convince her mother that this man had held her still with just one finger and his voice and his eyes burning her cheek? How could she make her mother understand that he had been horrible at the same time he had been kind? She couldn't remember anyone in her family ever telling her she was pretty.

She walked down to the dirt road that went into the orange grove at the end of their subdivision. She followed a narrow path between two rows of trees and let her mind go blank while her eyes rested on the symmetry of the grove. She found the spot to stand in to be the center of an X. Each way she looked, the trees lined up in diagonals for as far as she could see. She wouldn't tell her mother. She wouldn't tell Jack or Zeke.

She sat down on the ground where she had been standing and closed her eyes and then snuck her own finger under the elastic of her underpants and tried the back-and-forth motion. She scared herself. She didn't understand why she was doing this. Her legs itched and she was sure she was getting chiggers.

Ginny went to the tree hut after that only when she could go with Jack. The fear would grow in her as they started out until they reached the point where they could scan the whole clearing and she could see that the man wasn't there. Then she would burst through to elation and offer to race with Jack, or hoot and holler, or push him off-balance and knock him down with playful joy. Jack didn't seem to notice the difference in her. One day when they got home from school, he was ready to take off, but Ginny was supposed to peel the potatoes before she left. This had been carefully specified in a note from her mother. "Wait up," she said. "I can peel these in five minutes."

"I'll see you over at the hut," Jack said.

"Why don't you wait for me?"

"Why should I?"

Ginny shrugged. "Just because."

He took off without her, and all the while she peeled the potatoes, she thought about what she would say if she ran into the
man. And since she couldn't think of anything, she didn't go. She
went to her room and started on her homework instead. When
Jack came back, she was still working. He stuck his head into her
room. "How come you didn't show up?" he asked.

"I told you to wait up," she said.

"Spoilsport."

"I don't care."

"Shirley came," he said.

"So?"

"Well, we were waiting for you."

"So?"

"After you didn't show up, Zeke and I took turns kissing Shirley."

"You think I care?" Ginny said, lowering her eyes to her homework.

Jack gave her the face that said, "You think you're so great,
don't you," backed out of her doorway, and closed the door. She
picked up her papers and carefully stacked her school things beside the bed. Then she turned over and pushed her face into her
pillow and punched the mattress with her fists. The man had not
really made her stay. He had just acted as if she ought to. If only
she'd had the sense to move. Would he ever come again? Would
he think she would want him to? She realized she had not even
found out whether he owned the land.

She inspected the backs of her legs as she had done every day
since the old man. The chiggers still hadn't come out, and she
was almost positive they never would. She felt differently about
them now; their silence was hers. But she still felt like screaming:
It was my tree hut. Mine.

MARY BERGER

"I remember mostly the ominous quiet of those few moments, and my pulses pound."

Mary Berger (a pseudonym) was born in 1923 in Queens, New York. In her poem, "Summer Vacation/Fifty Years Ago," she describes a molestation that occurred half a century ago. She remembers the man well: "Like my family and me, he was vacationing at the tourist home during the Depression. He looked prosperous and respectable with gray hair and a moustache. He was clean and wore a jacket and knickers. Afterward, he was simply asked to leave the tourist home.

"The remainder of that day and the days that followed are a blank to me," Mary continues. "I did not question my parents' silence. My feelings of shame and embarrassment, which grew from that silence, were pushed away along with the dark memories of the experience."

As a child, Mary was shy and often alone. Her closest ties were with the women in the family. As she grew older and developed serious relationships with males, she found herself ambivalent about sex. "It was both an embarrassment and a joy," she writes, "always something I desired but never felt comfortable with. Fortunately I was never pressed to explain the loss of my virginity, and I have always felt I did lose it that day. I thought if my story were known, it would not be believed, or that it would seem like an excuse for attention. But why did I feel such guilt about being cheated out of my virginity!"

Mary lives with her husband in a small waterfront village on the East Coast. "I am happily married," she states. "I have had a full, though not always easy, life, doing all the things a woman does."

Summer Vacation/Fifty Years Ago

I ran down the hill
into the quiet of the woods
leaving the Tourist Home behind me.
The swing hanging from the tree
was too high to reach—
the old man stopped
lifted me, pushed me
back and forth, back and forth.
Counting to ten, I jumped
ran to be lifted again, again
we made a game of it. At first
he giggled with excitement
then his fingers were between my legs
rubbing, rough, hurting.
He stopped the swing
strange now, funny,
he crouched down in front of me
his hands on my knees
his face too close.
Everything was quiet, so quiet
except his breathing.
He lunged at me.
I jumped
knocking him over

scrambled up the hill, across the field
to where she was sitting with the other women.
Mother, that man was doing things.
Crying now, I showed her
like this and this.
She rushed me in the house—
behind me, I could hear my father swearing
above the voices of the other men.

We, I, never spoke of it again.

HUMMY

"The wounds are always there. Someone unknowingly kisses me while chewing spearmint-flavored gum, and they break open again and bleed."

Hummy was born in 1930 in Oswego, New York. When she was a few years old, her parents were divorced. New York law stated that because of the divorce she could not remain with her Native American tribe. She was given over to the custody of the court and placed in an orphanage. Thereafter she spent only three or four weeks a year with her mother.

When she was five years old, Hummy was brutally assaulted. She recounts this experience in "A Totally White World." As she recovered from her severe injuries, she often wished for death. "I wanted the Holy Mother to take me," she writes. "Without the constant care of my friend, Spring Flower, and the Medicine Woman, I wouldn't have recovered. I wouldn't have wanted to."

While Spring Flower gave her tender nursing, the Medicine Woman helped her regain strength in her arms and legs by building a weight-lifting machine for her. Because exercising on this machine was painful, Hummy was given an incentive. Every day the Medicine Woman made her rounds either in a buggy or in a sleigh pulled by her horse, Dora. "When you're strong enough," the Medicine Woman told Hummy, "you can drive Dora for me on my rounds." Hummy exercised and responded well to the Medicine Woman's moss packs and massages. Finally she was taken to the clinic to have her casts removed. As the doctor examined her, he exclaimed, "I can't believe how little atrophy there is!" "Atrophy" is still one of Hummy's favorite words.

Hummy was asexual until she was nineteen, when she became engaged to a man she had known all her life. Though they caressed, they were never sexually intimate. On the day they were to be married, he was killed en route to the chapel. She later married another man. "But it was three and a half months of counseling and patience on his part before we could have intercourse," she states. "He was a kind soul and a gentle lover. We had to make love with the lights on. I could not even sleep with him unless the lights were on."

Hummy lives in a small town in the Southwest as a successful businesswoman. She describes herself as "an asexual Amazon hoping to find love." She is still no closer to understanding the assault. "If I could give another title to the story," she concludes, "it would be 'Why?' "

A Totally White World

September 1935

I think to myself, what is that awful smell? It's like old Prestone, antifreeze. I groggily try to open my eyes. Oh, this is a totally white world. I can't seem to move my right arm. It's all painted white and seems to be in cement. My left arm is taped up with hoses running to it, like gas is being put into my arm, like putting gas in a car.

Where can I be? Is this a torture chamber? Did I get drunk like Apache Joe and get thrown in jail? What am I thinking? I don't drink except some of Spring's wine or applejack at a powwow.

No. I guess I must be dead. I wonder what I died of? I never thought it would be all white with the Sky People. I can't be dead—I have to pee. Such pain in my bowels. I have got to find a bathroom.

My head is really dizzy. I can't seem to lift my left leg. That's in cement, too. I'm going to throw up. Where can I do it? Out between the bars? What pain and fire in my stomach and bowels!

Oh, dear, Holy Mother, I can't seem to open my mouth. It's filled with wires. Here it comes. I just have to let it drool out of my mouth. I really have to find a bathroom.

"Peeja? Peeja!"

I hear a strange woman's voice say, "Go get the old woman so we can find out what she wants."

I hear soft footsteps coming toward me. They seem very familiar. Then I hear, "Hello, little Hummy." My heart smiles a big smile and I feel joy enter my body. I quickly say, "Thank you, Holy Mother, for sending me Spring Flower. Now I know everything will be all right."

"Spring, I have to go to the bathroom bad. I have bad cramps and I have to pee."

"Nurse, she has to go to the bathroom and she's thrown up here on the bed," Spring says.

"Tell her not to worry about the bathroom. She's all hooked up to bottles and her wastes go through tubes and are collected in the bottles under her bed. I will clean her up and bring some medicine for the pain and nausea."

"What am I doing here, Spring?" I ask her.

"Oh, honey, you took a terrible fall out of a big tree. You fell so hard that you tore yourself open. Part of your bowels were out of your body and your pelvic bone was crushed. Besides all that, you broke your jaw in four places. That's why your mouth is wired shut. Along with that, you broke nine ribs, your right arm is broken in three places, and the big bone in your left leg is broken. You have five cracks in your skull, and so many bruises.

"Miss Brockway and some of the children found you under the tree. You were unconscious. I want you to know, baby, you frightened ten years out of my soul in these past five days. My heart smiled when I heard you speak. It was nice to see you open at least one of your pretty brown eyes. Your nose looks like Suzie's pig's snout!

"Why are you speaking only in our tongue? It's important that you speak in the white tongue so that the nurses and doctors can help you with what you need. Besides, I have told you before, it's not polite to speak in our tongue when the people around can't understand what you are saying. You are in the white world now, so speak the white tongue."

Somewhere deep inside of me I really didn't want them to know what I was saying. "Won't Medicine Woman make me some nice moss packs to take this fire out of my body? I just know anything she would do would help. I know she could take away these awful pains. I hurt so bad in so many places, I don't know where I hurt most."

"Medicine Woman can't practice medicine here. She will take care of you when I take you to my house. The doctors and nurses take care of you here."

"Oh, dear, I'm going to be sick again."

"Turn your head to the side, dear," the nurse says. "Here, I'll put clean towels under your head. Now you'll feel a little bee sting in your right thigh. That's medicine for your pain and nausea."

Spring gently stroked my head and started to hum a lullaby. I began to feel drowsy and dreamy. I was sinking into a world covered with fuzz. I was just dozing off when a man's voice crashed into my dream. My body filled with terror. "Oh, Spring! Hide me, quick! Don't let them get me again!"

"Why are you shaking, child? Don't be afraid. I'm right here. I'll hold you. Well, maybe I can't hold you with all that paraphernalia you're hooked up to, but I'll stay close to you, Hummy. There, there, know I'm here. You can tell me all about what makes you feel so afraid."

"Oh, it was awful, Spring. I'll tell you the best I can remember:

"I was taking the shortcut behind the orphanage. I didn't want to be late for lunch washup. I saw these two fellows propped up against the tree by the old shed drinking out of bottles. The one guy named Floyd—he sometimes works around the orphanage—called over and said, "'Hey, Indian, will you take a note to Miss Durkey for me? If you will, I'll give you a quarter.'

"I said, 'Sure, I'm going there right now, but hurry—I don't want to be late.'

"I ran over to get the note, and that's when they grabbed me. I tried to yell, but the guy called Ernie put his hand over my mouth. They pushed me into the shed. I got my left hand free and scratched Floyd's face. He took my arm and smashed it over his knee. It sounded like someone splitting wood. It sent pain and fire up my arm and through my whole body.

"Floyd said, 'By God, if you can't hold on to that she-devil, we better tie her up.'

"Then they tied me between two posts, by wrists and ankles, spread out like you would stretch a hide to dry. Floyd stood over me and said, 'Toots, you're a bit feisty, but that's how I like my pussy.' He bent over and put his mouth on mine. He tasted terrible—like spearmint gum and whiskey. Oh, Spring, I don't think he ever took a bath. He smelled like the stinkiest sweat I ever smelled. I turned my head to spit. Floyd said, 'Don't you spit again or I'll smash you in your spitter.' He kept staring at me. Then he said, 'What a pretty little body. I'm going to give it the working over it deserves. You will know, Toots, what a real man is.'

"Then he took off his pants, walked over to me, and grabbed me by the hair. He pulled it so hard it made me squint. I thought he was going to pull it out by the roots. He shouted, 'Open your mouth, you filthy cunt. Here's a lollipop for you to suck on.'

"He pushed this piece of meat in my mouth that smelled like old pee and dirty socks. I didn't want that thing in my mouth, so I bit it. He yelled. Then he started hitting me in the face with his fists. My head seemed to snap back off my shoulders. My ears blew up. White stars flashed. I went off into blackness. A scream rose in my throat but was lost in blackness as he hit me again.

"I don't know how much time passed before I opened my eyes. I felt hard pebbles in my mouth. Some stuck to my gums. When I tried to spit them out, I realized they were my own teeth.

"He came toward me again and said, 'I don't like the way you stare at me with those filthy heathen eyes.' Then he hit me between the eyes. A hot pain filled my face, and my nose felt like it was being splintered all over. I sank back into darkness. . . .

"I can't talk any more about it now, Spring. I hurt too bad. If I can fall asleep, will you watch out for me?"

"Oh, she's awake," a man's voice said. I cringed, but Spring said, "It's all right, honey. This is one of your doctors."

"Could you answer some questions for me?" the doctor asked.

I spoke to Spring in our tongue and said I would try.

"Follow my finger with your eye without turning your head," he said.

I did it.

"Now squeeze my fingers."

I didn't like the idea of him touching me, but I did what he asked.

"She seems to understand English very well," he said.

"Yes, and she can also speak it very well if she has a mind to," Spring said.

"Can you tell me a little about your accident?" he asked.

I hurt too much. I said I was too tired to talk. I tried to fall asleep, but it was too frightening having him so near, even though his face looked kind.

I finally fell off into the world of fuzz, feeling very secure with

Spring holding my hand. Then I found the awful nightmare of Floyd hitting me again. I awakened crying, but was comforted to look into the deep, soft brown eyes of Spring. It was wonderful just looking at her beautiful, wise face.

"I know it's hard for you to talk about the accident, but it will be better for me to understand if you can tell me all about it, little darlin'."

"I'll try, Spring:

"I would wake up and there would be the two of them sitting across the room drinking out of these bottles. I asked if I could have a drink.

"Ernie said, 'Sure.' He got up and came over and poured some foul-tasting stuff in my mouth. All it did was make my mouth burn and taste bad. They both laughed.

"Floyd said, 'Can you get it up again, Ernie? I want you pumping me good when I get her cherry.'

"Then they came over near me. Ernie seemed to be doing something to Floyd. You know, like dogs do.

"Floyd said, 'Now you're cooking,' and they fell down on top of me.

"Floyd said, 'Now I'm going to give this slut what she deserves.'

"He shoved something between my legs that felt like a knife cutting me open, splitting me apart. He kept pushing and pushing and pushing, slamming me into the floor. I felt like I was being crushed and torn apart at the same time. The pain was so bad, I must have passed out. I woke up gagging and throwing up.

"Floyd yelled at Ernie, 'Go come in her face so I can watch.' Through the haze of Floyd slamming my body into the floor, I felt a hot wetness on my face. Floyd yelled something. Then he stopped pushing. I kept throwing up with the pain and nausea. Finally I passed out.

"I was half awake when I heard Ernie say, 'I'm going outside to take a shit.'

"Floyd said, 'Why don't you shit on that outhouse Indian over there?'

"'I can't do that,' Ernie said.

"'I'll show you how to do it, Ernie.'

"Floyd came over to me, looked down, and said, 'Listen, you god damn bunch of garbage. You want a drink? Well, here's one.' Then he peed in my face.

"'That piss will get some of the rotten Indian smell off you. This will help, too.' He squatted over me and crapped on my stomach.

"I tried to roll over and dump it off, but I was tied too tightly. Then he put his butt in my face and said, 'Lick me off.'

"The stink was so horrible, I just vomited on him.

"Oh, how I prayed for Mother Death to come and take me to the Sky People. I guess I smelled so bad even she didn't want me. I just passed out with the pain.

"I woke up again when they were turning me over on my stomach. Floyd said, 'Look, Ernie, you can tell a real man got her cherry. Look at all the red flowing.'

"When they rolled me over, I screamed as loud as I could. Floyd kicked my left leg so hard, I could hear it crunch. 'Shut up, you stinking slut,' he said.

"The pain was so bad, I must have fainted.

"I half woke up to feel myself being pushed into the floor. Sharp pains were flooding my stomach and groin. Oh, how I begged the Holy Mother to take me. The slamming and the pain just wouldn't let up.

"'Jesus, Floyd, you better stop. You're turning her inside out. Hey, Floyd, I think she's had it,' Ernie said.

"'I'm getting sick of her anyway. Roll her over,' Floyd said.

"I didn't move. I played I was asleep. Then he kicked me in the ribs. The cracking sound and fiery pain came at the same time. I felt like I would never breathe again. I didn't know where I was hurting worst.

"'God, Floyd, I think you killed her,' Ernie said.

"'Oh, that god damn pussy couldn't take a real man,' Floyd said. 'We'll come back and burn it down after dark. They'll think she fell asleep in here and accidentally tipped over the lantern. We better untie her so it will look like she was asleep.'

"I didn't move. It hurt too bad to breathe deeply, so I took a little breath. I didn't move. I was trying to keep my head clear so I could get out of there. I waited a long time after I heard their voices and footsteps fade away.

"Oh, I was so dizzy when I raised my head that I got sick to my stomach again. It was so hard to get up over the pain, to get my thoughts together. I knew I had to get out of there. I felt around and found my clothes. I struggled to get my panties on and to get the parts of me that were hanging out of me into my panties. I don't know how long that took, because I kept getting dizzy and passing out. I decided that I wouldn't try to put on the rest of my clothes. I just tied them around my neck.

"I dragged myself for a long time, passing in and out of blackness. I kept going because I knew I didn't want to burn. Finally I was outside. I could hear the peepers and knew that's where there was water. I couldn't burn where there was water. I don't know how long or how far I dragged myself, but finally I was by the water. I went into the water, which seemed to wake me up a little. Then I knew I had to clean myself. I would wash and wash myself as long as I could stay awake. My face would fall into the water. I would rise back up choking and gasping. Pain tore all through my body. I wanted to keep my head underwater forever.

"I came to some cattails and crawled up on them. They seemed to keep me from sinking. I heard men's voices off in the distance. I smelled smoke. I heard the cracking of fire. I didn't move or look to see where it was. I was trying very hard not to move or moan when I breathed.

"A long time passed. Then there were the regular night

sounds. I hurt so bad that I was glad when I drifted off into blackness.

"The next thing I remember was Mother Sun warming me. I was shivering so hard I couldn't think. The shivering just seemed to make the pain worse. I tried to open my eyes, and finally I was able to see out of my left one. I saw the orphanage rooftop off in the distance, so I started crawling toward it. I don't remember anything after that except crawling and praying to Mother Death to please take me. Would I ever be clean again? I didn't feel I was worth anything, and I didn't think I ever would be if I lived."

One day I woke up to hear Spring Flower speaking with the doctor. I could tell by the sound of her voice that she was angry.

"They need to be brought to justice," she said.

The doctor said, "She would have to identify them. It would be her word, a five-year-old Indian child against two adult white men. She has suffered enough. I don't think you could ever bring it to trial."

"Doctor, you're misunderstanding me," Spring Flower said. "I definitely do not want her involved in any way. I just want to know where they can be located. You can help me or not. These men will be found and will be treated accordingly. We, too, have our justice."

JEAN ALEXANDER

"One has to try to feel hopeful that, as awareness increases, perhaps these terrible crimes against children will lessen. However, my last question still stands."

Jean Alexander was born in England in the Thirties and spent much of her childhood in Scotland with her mother's relatives. The incident she describes in "Letter to a Soldier" came to be written because of two events in her life that coincided: an unpleasant incident with a lover that left her feeling, in her words, "bruised, self-condemning, and spiritually raped," and hearing the phrase "rope swing" at a poetry reading. The phrase evoked in her an overwhelming sadness, but she was not sure why.

The morning after the poetry reading, Jean could not work as usual in her potter's studio and sat listlessly. "I lit a fire in the living room and just sat in front of it, staring into the flames," she writes. "I leaned forward to poke a log and suddenly found myself crying like a heartbroken child and beating the poker against the grate again and again."

Shortly after this, Jean was able to complete the catharsis by writing the story. "It not only helped rid me of that half-submerged childhood ghost," she says, "but it was also the painful beginning of a new way of looking at myself and my relationships with men."

Jean considers herself lucky in that the incident did not cause her irreparable psychological damage. At the present time, she lives contentedly in Sussex, England, as a crafts coordinator at a home for the chronically disabled. "Yet the scars were there," she

points out, "and the memory of the crushing fear and the uncom-
prehending guilt." She concludes: "The anger remains—that gen-
erations of children have been sexually used, abused, scarred, and
even murdered, and that it continues in spite of all our social
'progress.'"

Letter to a Soldier

There are some oak trees in the meadow by the river. They are
immense, gnarled and green-mossed, said in legend to be the only
trees left standing when Macduff hewed Birnam Wood and
marched his men in their greenwood disguises upon Macbeth.

We—that is, my cousin Jimmy and I—weren't thinking of history that day. Do you remember two small children swinging on a
rope hung from one of the ancient, massive branches? The end of
the rope was knotted into a heavy, bristly, uncomfortable lump
that chafed my bottom and scratched my legs. You watched us
swing for a time, then you said, nodding your head toward me,
"Come on, I'll make you a proper swing out of wood."

I went with you up the narrow path to the old mansion your
regiment had taken over, and you took my hand as we climbed
the steep bank. Your hand was very big, and warm. I remember it
felt nice. Grandpa had big, strong, warm hands, too, stained and
checked with the leather he worked with every day, and the tobacco he rolled between his thickened fingers, and the live coals
he used to light his pipe—but he wasn't much for holding hands.
So your hand felt nice.

At the top of the bank, we went through the shrubbery that
ringed the once-elegant circular lawn. I remember a mock-orange
bush with waxy white blossoms, heavy sensual scent. Usually as I
passed that bush I'd snap off a sprig to take to my grandmother,

but I didn't that day because I was afraid you'd tell me off for
stealing your flowers. We passed the dilapidated summerhouse
and crossed the shaggy, daisy-sparkled lawn. You explained that
you were alone, as you were the cook today and had to stay. Your
tools were in the house, you said. Come upstairs.

I followed you up the wide staircase. There were no banisters.
Evacuees from the slums of Glasgow, who had lived in the house
before the soldiers came, had torn them down to use as firewood,
and there were gaping plaster wounds in the dark oak paneling of
the walls. Your room was small and rather bare. A narrow bed,
gray blankets. You fetched some wood and some tools, and sat
straddle-legged on a low stool as you worked. It was then I noticed
it. The front of your khaki trousers was open, and "it" hung like a
limp maggot between your legs. You looked at me strangely then,
and you said, "I'll give you sixpence for sweeties if you'll take
down your knickers."

A sixpenny poke of sweeties—for what? In fear, I turned to the
door. You held my arm tightly and sat me on your knee, while
your other hand groped under my skirt and I heard my underwear
tearing and felt the cruel hardness of your fingers on my sex. I
jerked myself free somehow and stumbled down the stairs, and as
I ran through the front door, I heard you hiss, "Don't you tell!"

Jimmy sulked all the way home to my grandmother's house. He
hadn't wanted to leave his game so soon.

I didn't tell granny about you. I told her I'd torn my knickers
climbing a tree, and she was angry, until she noticed the deep
scratches your nails had left on my legs. Then she said, "Lord,
lassie, you puir wee thing," and daubed me with iodine, which
had a vengeful sting to it.

Suddenly today I am remembering you, soldier, and crying.
Crying for that five-year-old child, worth only a sixpenny poke of
sweeties to you. Crying for God knows how many other innocent
little cunts. Where are you now, soldier? Some dark heart in me
hopes you died choking on your own blood in the cold muck of

war. No. That's not what I wish. I hope your balls were torn and splattered and that long, maggoty "it" was blown from between your legs. No. I can't wish that either. Damn you, why can't I wish for your hurt, your mutilation? What did you care for mine? How many children? . . . How many sixpences?

JENNIFER MEYER

"Walking down dark streets at night, a confidence hums round my body like a shield."

Jennifer Meyer was born in 1954 in Jonesboro, Arkansas. Three years before the incident described in "Crossing the Fence," Jennifer was molested in a dressmaker's shop in Italy. While hemming Jennifer's coat, the tailor reached into her underwear even as Jennifer's mother and sister sat a few yards away. Jennifer did not react in any way, feeling that the embarrassment of a scene would be more difficult to endure than the act itself.

During the following three years, she found an inner strength manifesting itself in open, expressed anger. "If my mother lost her quiet, docile, devoted daughter," she writes, "if, instead, she found living in her house an angry, rebellious, sharp-tongued teen-ager, she had no reason to grieve." Jennifer feels that learning to "talk back" was an important part of her transition into becoming an assertive adult.

Two years after the second incident, Jennifer was threatened again. A man pushed her up against a tree and told her he intended to rape her. "I bored my gaze beyond his pupils and, for what seemed like minutes, I didn't breathe," she writes. "'No, you're not,' I finally said in a sturdy whisper." The man withdrew without harming her.

Jennifer reveals a fantasy she often has: "I'm walking alone down a dark street at night; a passing man makes a rude remark and moves into my path. I lunge toward him, shouting, 'I've been

254

wanting an excuse to kill someone tonight!'" She continues: "The
greatness of this angry strength rising up unsolicited frightens
even me. It's not surprising that no one has ever given me the
chance to carry out this fantasy."

Crossing the Fence

To get to my high school, I walked through the woods behind our
house, over the gate to the horse pasture, around the pond, over
another gate, and up a red dust road. Sometimes I met my friend
Debbie at the bottom of the hill and trekked across the field with
her, but lately she'd given up on me because I was always late.

This was one of my "worst years," as my mother would later
refer to it, and there was rarely a morning I wasn't detained by a
fight with my parents. When the homeroom bell rang at school
and everyone else was grimacing in the direction of the flag while
the scratchy sounds of the national anthem wallowed in varying
speeds over the loudspeaker, I was usually slamming the door to
my bedroom.

The morning arguments were always over my appearance. I
was trying my hardest to be a hippie, and my parents found almost everything about me appalling. At breakfast they would
threaten to keep me home from school if I wouldn't change my
clothes. If I shrugged my shoulders and complied without protest,
they'd instantly change tack and tell me I had to go.

Finally I would stomp loudly to my bedroom, blowing long,
exasperated sighs through my teeth like a steam iron. Minutes
later I would appear in a skirt and blouse, not quite matching, but
conspicuously unoffending. "Private Meyer reporting for inspec-
tion, *sir!*" I would snap at my father with a nasty salute. ("Just
asking to be slapped," my mother would cry.) My father would

mumble resentful approval of my attire, and I would rush out the door with a slam.

One day in spring, I had just crossed the fence when I heard a rustling in the bushes to my left. I looked up to see a man, naked from the waist down. He was watching me, but I pretended not to see him. I kept on walking and didn't dare look back.

"Hey, wait," he said. I considered running but decided it was best not to initiate a race. "Hey, girl," he continued, "come here. Come suck me. Come suck my cock."

I pretended to be deaf and hastened my pace to a stiff-legged trot. I scanned the field for help. On the far side of the pasture, I saw a boy hastily climbing the fence. I wondered whether he was rushing because he was late for school or because he, too, had seen this man. As I debated whether or not to call out, the boy disappeared down the road.

I heard the man's feet crushing the weeds behind me and I glanced back to see him getting closer. Penis in hand, he shouted a string of lewd suggestions. My face grew hot and my heart was pounding, but I judged the remaining distance of the pasture and knew I wouldn't make it if he chased me. His voice grew closer, and fear clutched at my chest.

Suddenly I spun on my heels and faced the man. He stumbled awkwardly to a stop and looked at me dumbly. He was short and overweight. His blond hair was slicked down over part of his forehead. He wore a blue mechanic's shirt with a patch that said "SHELL, Hi—Bob." Standing frozen in the middle of a step, his weight on the forward foot, he looked ridiculous. My fear began to evaporate and I might have laughed if I hadn't been trying so hard to be vicious.

"Get out of here," I growled, clenching my fists to hide the trembling.

He hesitated, then, inching forward, said, "Here, touch it. Look."

I did the only thing I could think of: I shouted, without pause and as loud as I could, every obscenity I had ever heard. I watched his face file through a dozen expressions, unable to find the right one, as I flung the words at him like bullets. "Leave me alone!"

I stood panting, fists still clenched. He had let go his grasp on himself and his penis now hung hideously limp against the white of his thighs. I glanced at it with disgust, then bored my eyes fiercely into his.

I turned and walked away, listening carefully for the sound of his feet behind me. When I was sure he wasn't following me, my chest relaxed and I could breathe. All that was left of the fear was the sweat under my bangs. I walked fast, my arms swinging, and I grinned to myself.

Climbing the gate, I stopped and looked back across the field. The man scurried along the row of trees near the fence, hopping painfully through the bed of cockleburs.

"Ha!" I bellowed, the cry rising from my belly like a cannonball and echoing over the pond. The man quickly dodged behind a tree. I straddled the gate, gloating, elated. I felt unconquerable. I lifted my face to the sky and I laughed triumphantly. My laughing echoed in the hills and I felt stronger than I ever knew I was. I jumped down to the dirt road and sprinted the rest of the way to school.

Afterword

My heart is moved by all I cannot save: so much has been destroyed
I have to cast my lot with those who age after age, perversely,
with no extraordinary power, reconstitute the world.

—Adrienne Rich

As I sat down to write this Afterword, I re-read the Introduction
I wrote a decade ago. The Introduction is less than forty pages. It
took me three years to write. In the process I was re-thinking
everything I had ever thought about the world, everything I had
assumed to be true—and suddenly found out was not. Those three
years were life-changing: disturbing, exciting, painful, and honest.
I found out more about "man's inhumanity to man"—and especially to women and children—than I had ever imagined could be
true. I wept. I raged. I searched for meaning.

Today, ten years later, I am still weeping, raging, and searching
for meaning. I'm also loving. My work for these years has been to
be a witness to survivors' healing. And as a witness, what I found
in my heart, along with the grief and fury, was love. And respect.
And gratitude for such honesty and trust.

When I began this work I knew nothing about the healing
process. Indeed, I didn't even think in those terms. I didn't start
with an idea that survivors were damaged and it was my job to "fix"
them. I came, instead, as a human being, moved by the experiences
of other human beings—and by the ways they survived those experiences. To my surprise, this turned out to be healing.

One of the most dramatic examples of this occurred while we
were preparing biographical notes for the contributors to *I Never
Told Anyone*. We had written, asking them to tell us a little about
their process of healing from the abuse, and one woman, whose

258

poem described an event that had occurred fifty years previously, wrote back saying that she had been in therapy for twenty years with several different therapists, but had never discussed the abuse. After getting our inquiry, she took the poem to her therapist and said she wanted to talk about it—for the first time in her life.

Unintentionally, we were discovering the elements of the healing process. We were supporting women to break the silence, to understand that it wasn't their fault, to be angry, to grieve, to believe that it mattered that they were abused. We were offering our own outrage, our respect, and our belief in their stories. We were caring, in a very simple, straightforward way. And it was meaningful. It was healing.

When *I Never Told Anyone* was completed, I expected its publication to be the end of my involvement with the issue of child sexual abuse. I had begun working on it several months after the birth of my first child, a daughter, and in retrospect it seems clear to me that it was, in part, my attempt to make the world a safer place for her. When the book was done I thought that was that. I'd made my contribution and I could return to my own writing and teaching.

But sometimes we are led in ways we never consciously intend, and this is what happened for me. Because there was a need for a safe, supportive space in which survivors of child sexual abuse could share their experiences, I began offering workshops for survivors. And as these survivors taught me more about the healing process, I amassed a great deal of information that other survivors needed, culminating five years later in *The Courage to Heal: A Guide for Women Survivors of Child Sexual Abuse*, which I coauthored with Laura Davis.

For over a decade, then, my work has centered around helping individual survivors to heal from child sexual abuse. This has been the most inspiring work I can imagine having done; the rewards have been great. I have had the pleasure of watching survivors move through despair into creative, satisfying lives. I have had the privilege of taking a small part in making that happen. And for myself, I have learned an enormous amount about courage, change, healing, goodness, and the power of love.

And so now I come to this place of reflection—looking back at the work that's been done and the work there is still to do.

In the years since *I Never Told Anyone* was published, survivors of child sexual abuse have gone from being single, brave voices to being a strong and vital community, a national force. Hundreds of thousands of survivors have entered into a healing process in a conscious and determined way. It has been a decade of massive personal recovery. Following the example of women who were raped, survivors of child sexual abuse have joined in large numbers to speak out about the abuse they suffered, to acknowledge that it was never their fault, to assert their right to be outraged, and to combine their intelligence, compassion, and creativity to heal themselves and each other. By the thousands, and hundreds of thousands, they are reclaiming their lives, refusing to be victims, refusing to remain powerless.

Clearly, we've broken the silence. In newspapers and magazines, on the radio and television, people are acknowledging the sexual abuse of children. There is support now. All over the country there are survivors' groups: self-help groups, 12-step groups, therapy groups, workshops, and conferences. There are newsletters, books, videos, cassettes, legal resources. Although the services available are still not accessible enough and not of consistently high quality, a beginning has been made. Professionals now know much more about how to help survivors heal.

Yet, as in the beginning, it is the survivors who are the experts. When I lead training seminars for people who provide services for survivors, I often ask, "How many people went to schools that offered a major program in working with survivors of child sexual abuse?" Out of a group of five hundred professionals, usually it's none. Then I ask how many have had a substantial course—at least one semester long? Usually a few. How many have had at least some

kind of a course? Maybe ten percent. Surely we, as service providers, have not learned about how to work with survivors from our
academic training.

We learned from survivors themselves. This was, and continues
to be, a grass-roots movement. It grew out of our consciousness as
women and as feminists. Its foundations were the rape crisis movement, take back the night groups, self-defense classes, women's
centers, consciousness-raising groups. It grew out of women's politics and our accurate understanding that "the personal is political."

None of us suffers in a vacuum. To forget that child sexual abuse
occurs in a social and political context leaves us ignorantly vulnerable.

We have come a long way in the past decade. The successes are
great. Personally, I think of all the women I know who are alive and
healing, who might otherwise have given up and died. And I think
of all the women I've never met who are protecting their children,
now that they have faced their own abuse and can see and react
responsibly. I think of the women—and men—who are not going
on to abuse children because they have faced their own abuse and
are working through their own healing. I think of all those who have
been able to say the abuse stops here.

In the past decade, men have begun to acknowledge the sexual
abuse they suffered as children. Rather than continue to perpetuate
the tough stereotype of what being a real man is, male survivors
have begun to share their stories of victimization—of pain, fear,
and the outrage that comes from loving their vulnerable young
selves. Men are joining their voices with those of women to grieve,
change, heal, and create a safer world.

We've begun to face issues we dared not confront before. Were
I editing *I Never Told Anyone* today, more stories of abuse by
women would be included. Although there is one example here of
abuse by a grandmother, we received very few submissions of writing by women abused by women. There has been an exceptionally
strong taboo against talking about female perpetrators.

Although the bulk of sexual abuse is clearly perpetrated by men, substantial numbers of women abuse, and when they do, they are capable of the same brutality as men. This has been especially hard for me to face. I have wanted to believe that women, though they sometimes do not protect their children, are not actually the abusers themselves. But this is an illusion. And though disillusionment is painful, until we face the truth, we cannot protect the children abused by women or help the survivors of such abuse to heal.

Change is happening. It is too slow. It is not enough. But it still counts. I think of the words of Gandhi: "Almost anything you do will be insignificant, but it is very important that you do it." And so we make progress.

Children are benefitting from child safety and abuse prevention courses. They are being taught to tell and to tell again if they're not listened to. They are being taught that no one has the right to abuse them, that they have the right to their own bodies, to control who touches them and how. And children are beginning to tell.

Yet when children *do* tell, they are still not always believed. And when the abuse is reported, often there is not an adequate response. Child Protective Services are overloaded and cannot respond effectively to the calls they receive. There aren't adequate foster homes for children whose parents are abusive or neglectful. Often the abuse can't be proved, and the child isn't considered credible. Cases don't come to trial. Perpetrators get off lightly. Prosecutors don't have the experience or knowledge to conduct a case for a successful verdict.

Yet, there have been some impressive successes in the legal arena. In June 1990, the Supreme Court ruled that children do not have to face their abusers in court. Using videotaping, the child can be spared the further trauma of a face-to-face meeting with the abuser.

In many states survivors are lobbying to change the statute of limitations so that they can sue their perpetrators in civil court when they have the strength and resources to do so, even if it's many years after the abuse. The principle of delayed discovery is being used to enable the survivor to sue as an adult, the antecedent being that—as in other personal injury cases—the damage is not necessarily clear at the time of injury. Survivors are winning these suits, and in some cases the verdicts are substantial.

There is also backlash. As survivors have gotten stronger and more outspoken, as non-abusive parents have gotten more aggressive about protecting their children, there's been a backlash from abusers and those who want to maintain the *status quo*. Mothers who've tried to keep their children safe from abusive fathers have been accused of lying just to maintain custody. They've been accused of using the issue as a way to manipulate or get back at a divorced husband. Mothers have been forced to go underground with their children, or to send their children underground to protect them from sexually abusive fathers. Mothers have gone to jail rather than hand their children over to abusive fathers.

The fact that mothers are going to such lengths to protect their children is at once both a triumph—a glorious triumph of sane, fierce, mother-love—and a crime that such action should be necessary in our legal system, which continues to be so protective of abusers and unprotective of children. And of course, children are still being abused. Even as we work so hard to heal, more children are abused every day and will also need to do all that long arduous work of healing. All our progress has not made children safe.

As I wrote a decade ago, we live in a world which condones and enables child sexual abuse. Child sexual abuse is not an aberrant behavior in our society, but one which conforms to our beliefs, expectations, and laws. Until there is respect for all people, not just the ones with power, but everyone, then we are not going to have impressive success in stopping child sexual abuse.

The connections between our society's values, institutions, and priorities and child sexual abuse become exceedingly clear when we look at the extremes of abuse, such as ritual or cult abuse. Survivors of ritual abuse have begun to tell their stories of physical, sexual, psychological, and spiritual torture by organized groups. These stories are horrific—and true.

Until recently very few survivors of ritual abuse dared to tell anyone what had happened to them for fear—well-justified—that they would be labeled crazy, lying, or both. Also, the admonitions and threats not to tell are so severe that many survivors find it terrifying to talk about the abuse. But now organizations are working to share information and healing resources, as well as to address the criminal justice and prevention aspects of such abuse.

This abuse has been allowed to go on, virtually unhampered, because the legal system, organized religion, the medical establishment, and others in positions of power have been either involved or paid off by these groups. The child pornography industry is linked with such cults in that they film abuse and torture, and then they sell it. Children are also supplied by cults for prostitution, and the revenue increases. This is a multi-billion-dollar business. If we are to achieve real and substantial progress in protecting children against abuse, we must effect political and social change.

When the chief of police is in on abusing children, the criminal justice system isn't going to work too well in that city. When the judge is part of a cult, Child Protective Services isn't going to get very far. When the chief of staff at the hospital patches up children and hushes up the abuse for a pay-off, or because he's a pedophile himself, proof of abuse is going to be hard to document.

As Alice Walker said, "I'm an activist. It pays the rent for being on the planet." We all owe it. We need to work actively for a world that respects life more than it respects money, power, and the rights of abusers to devastate children.

So there has been progress, but it is not enough. Not nearly enough. I tell myself it is unrealistic to expect more. It has been only a decade—such a short time—a very short time to change consciousness, to change the patterns of centuries. I tell myself that these changes will lead to more changes, that the tide is turning and will keep on turning for the better. But it's going to take more than hope and good intentions. There is still enormous work to be done.

When I look at all that's happened positively, I can feel optimistic. When I look at how many children are still being abused and how woefully inadequate our society is in responding compassionately and furiously to that abuse, I can feel pessimistic. But mostly I don't engage too much in either of these responses. I simply keep on doing the work. I am inspired by a quote from Danilo Dolci, the Italian poet, educator, and non-violent activist:

> *There are moments when things go well and one feels encouraged. There are difficult moments and one feels overwhelmed. But it's senseless to speak of optimism or pessimism. The only important thing is to know that if one works well in a potato field, the potatoes will grow. If one works well among men [and women], they will grow— that's reality. The rest is smoke. It's important to know that words don't move mountains. Work, exacting work, moves mountains.*

Some words, of course, are a part of the work, such as words that break the silence around child sexual abuse. But the point here is that we don't have to question whether things can get better, whether we can be effective in stopping child sexual abuse and helping survivors to heal. Of course we can. It is inevitable that as individual survivors heal in larger numbers, there will be far-reaching effects even beyond our imaginations. The energy that has been bound up in simply coping, trying to live under the burdens of the damage of the abuse, becomes freed, available. It is a huge reservoir of energy that can be turned to any purpose.

Each survivor's own healing comes first. That is a necessity. But it cannot stop there. It is not enough for survivors to heal only themselves. It is not enough for service providers to focus only on helping individuals to heal. And it is not enough for those of us who are not survivors to sit back, seeing all the exposure on television, in the newspapers and books, and assume that it's being taken care of, to assume that the world is changing for the good and doesn't need our help. It does. It's critical that we each do our part to work for a world in which there is respect, even reverence, for life.

Resources

ORGANIZATIONS

HEALING HEARTS, 1515 Webster St., Oakland, CA 94612, (415) 465-3890.
Healing Hearts is a service organization for adult survivors of ritual abuse. They offer a newsletter, institutes, and conferences.

INCEST RESOURCES, INC. Cambridge Women's Center, 46 Pleasant St., Cambridge, MA 02139, (617) 354-8807.
Incest Resources publishes excellent low-cost literature on incest-related topics and offers a referral service.

LOOKING UP, P.O. Box K, Augusta, ME 04330, (207) 626-3402.
Looking Up provides referrals, low-cost conferences, workshops, and wilderness trips.

PARENTS UNITED (Adults Molested As Children United), P.O. Box 952, San Jose, CA 95108, (408) 280-5055.
Parents United works with the whole family when incest occurs, with a focus on reconciliation. They also sponsor AMAC groups for adult survivors. In many cases, AMACs are urged to participate in groups with perpetrators. Some survivors find these groups a great way to get in touch with anger, but others feel forced into a philosophy of treatment they don't believe in or want.

PLEA (Prevention, Leadership, Education and Assistance). PLEA serves nonoffending male survivors of sexual, physical, and emotional abuse. For information, contact Hank Estrada, Box 22, West Zia Rd, Santa Fe, NM 87505, (505) 982-9184

SCAP (Survivors of Childhood Abuse Program), 1345 El Centro Ave., P.O. Box 630, Hollywood, CA 90028.
Provides networking, training, consultation, advocacy, resources, and public education on abuse-related issues. For referrals and information, call their National Childhood Abuse Hotline: (800) 422-4453.

Survivors of Incest Anonymous, P.O. Box 21817, Baltimore, MD 21222, (301) 282-3400.
A 12-step recovery program for survivors of child sexual abuse that provides meetings in many cities nationally. They publish excellent literature on sexual abuse and recovery.

The Safer Society Program, Shoreham Depot Rd., RR1, Box 24-B, Orwell, VT 05760, (802) 897-7541.
The Safer Society Program maintains national lists of agencies and individuals who provide assessment and treatment for sexual abuse victims and offenders. Their excellent collection of publications includes many books of interest to adult survivors.

12-Step Programs: Alcoholics Anonymous, Narcotics Anonymous, Al-Anon, Adult Children of Alcoholics, Incest Survivors Anonymous, Sex and Love Addicts Anonymous, Overeaters Anonymous, Gamblers Anonymous, Debtors Anonymous, and others are national organizations which provide free, confidential meetings. For information on meetings in your area, check the phone book for local chapter offices, or contact any social service agency or religious institution for referrals.

VOICES in Action, Inc., P.O. Box 148309, Chicago, IL 60614.
A national self-help network for survivors and "pro-survivors" (partners and friends of survivors), VOICES offers referrals, an annual conference, a newsletter, and special-interest support groups.

BOOKS

Sexual Abuse

BAER, EUAN, WITH PETER DIMOCK. *Adults Molested as Children: A Survivor's Manual for Women and Men.* Orwell, VT: Safer Society Press, 1988.
A simple, straightforward approach to healing. (To order, send $12.95 to Safer Society Press, Shoreham Depot Rd., RR #1, Box 24-B, Orwell, VT 05760-9756.)

BASS, ELLEN, AND LAURA DAVIS. *The Courage to Heal: A Guide for Women Survivors of Child Sexual Abuse.* New York: Harper & Row, 1988.
An inspiring, comprehensive guide. (Also available on audiocassette.)

BLUME, E. SUE. *Secret Survivors: Uncovering Incest and Its Aftereffects in Women.* New York: John Wiley & Sons, 1989.
Supportive, validating, and healing.

BRADY, KATHERINE. *Father's Days: A True Story of Incest.* New York: Dell, 1979.
A first-person account of father-daughter incest.

BRIERE, JOHN. *Therapy for Adults Molested As Children: Beyond Survival.* New York: Springer Publishing, 1989.
A sensible guide for therapists.

BUTLER, SANDRA. *Conspiracy of Silence: The Trauma of Incest.* San Francisco: Volcano Press, 1985 (updated).
A classic. Feminist analysis of child sexual abuse.

COURTOIS, CHRISTINE. *Healing the Incest Wound: Adult Survivors in Therapy.* New York: W. W. Norton, 1988.
A feminist psychologist writes a useful guidebook for therapists on healing.

DANICA, ELLY. *Don't: A Woman's Word. A Personal Chronicle of Child-hood Incest and Adult Recovery.* San Francisco: Cleis Press, 1988. Horrifying, vivid, and poetic.

DONAFORTE, LAURA. *I Remembered Myself: The Journal of a Survivor of Childhood Sexual Abuse.* Self-published, 1982. The day-to-day struggles, pain, and triumphs of healing.

EVERT, KATHY, AND INIE BIJKERK. *When You're Ready: A Woman's Healing from Childhood Physical and Sexual Abuse by Her Mother.* Walnut Creek, CA: Launch Press, 1988. A powerful resource for women molested by their mothers.

FINKELHOR, DAVID. *Sexually Victimized Children.* New York: The Free Press, 1979. Combines survivors' accounts with research data in a readable style. *Child Sexual Abuse: New Theory and Research* is the follow-up.

FORTUNE, MARIE M. *Sexual Violence: The Unmentionable Sin: An Ethi-cal and Pastoral Perspective.* New York: Pilgrim Press, 1983. Written from a Christian and feminist point of view.

GIL, ELIANA. *Outgrowing the Pain: A Book for and about Adults Abused as Children.* San Francisco: Launch Press, 1983. A helpful place to begin. Her second book, *Treatment of Adult Survivors of Child Sexual Abuse,* is a practical guide for mental health professionals.

HERMAN, JUDITH. *Father-Daughter Incest.* Cambridge: Harvard Univer-sity Press, 1981. Well-written, well-researched, from a feminist perspective.

KAHANER, LARRY. *Cults That Kill.* New York: Warner Books, 1988. Series of interviews focusing on cults, especially satanic.

LEW, MIKE. *Victims No Longer: Men Recovering from Incest and Other Sexual Child Abuse.* New York: Harper & Row, 1990. Solid, clear, warm information and encouragement.

MALTZ, WENDY, AND BEVERLY HOLMAN. *Incest and Sexuality: A Guide to Understanding and Healing.* Lexington, MA: Lexington Books, 1987.
An excellent resource for working through sexual (and other) problems. Also read the comprehensive *The Sexual Healing Journey.* New York: HarperCollins, forthcoming 1991.

McNARON, TONI, AND YARROW MORGAN. *Voices in the Night: Women Speaking About Incest.* Minneapolis: Cleis Press, 1982.
Includes mother-daughter incest.

MILLER, ALICE. *Thou Shalt Not Be Aware: Society's Betrayal of the Child.* New York: New American Library, 1986.
Required reading for every therapist. Miller has written two other excellent books: *The Drama of the Gifted Child* and *For Your Own Good: Hidden Cruelty in Child-rearing and the Roots of Violence.*

MORRIS, MICHELLE. *If I Should Die Before I Wake.* New York: Dell, 1982.
A harrowing fictional account of incest.

POSTON, CAROL, AND KAREN LISON. *Reclaiming Our Lives: Hope for Adult Survivors of Incest.* Boston: Little Brown, 1989.
Down-to-earth help for women survivors.

PUTNAM, FRANK W. *Diagnosis & Treatment of Multiple Personality Disorder.* New York: The Guilford Press, 1989.
The best overview.

RANDALL, MARGARET. *This Is About Incest.* Ithaca: Firebrand Books, 1987.
Using words and photography, Margaret Randall documents her healing.

RUSH, FLORENCE. *The Best Kept Secret: Sexual Abuse of Children.* Englewood Cliffs: Prentice-Hall, 1980.
An excellent feminist analysis of child sexual abuse from biblical times to Freud to the present.

RUSSELL, DIANA. *The Secret Trauma: Incest in the Lives of Girls and Women.* New York: Basic Books, 1986.
With comprehensive research, this book validates the damage of incest.

SISK, SHEILA, AND CHARLOTTE FOSTER HOFFMAN. *Inside Scars: Incest Recovery as Told by a Survivor and Her Therapist.* Gainsville, FL: Pandora Press, 1987.
A first-person account of healing.

SMITH, MICHELLE, AND LAURENCE PAZDER. *Michelle Remembers.* New York: Pocket Books, 1980.
A ritual abuse survivor writes with her therapist about healing.

TERRY, MOREY. *The Ultimate Evil.* New York: Dolphin, 1987.
Written by an investigative reporter, this account of the trial of David Berkowitz, the "Son of Sam," includes information about satanic cults and ritual abuse.

WHITE, LOUISE. *The Obsidian Mirror: An Adult Healing from Incest.* Seattle: Seal Press, 1988.
A powerfully written description of the healing process.

WOITITZ, JANET. *Healing Your Sexual Self.* Deerfield Beach, FL: Health Communication, 1989.
Focuses on identifying sexual abuse and recognizing its long-term effects.

For Parents

COLAO, FLORA, AND TAMAR HOSANSKY. *Your Children Should Know.* New York: Berkeley Books, 1983.
A top resource book for parents. Why, how, and when to talk to your children. What to do if assault occurs. Teaching children to be powerful.

HAGANS, KATHRYN, AND JOYCE CASE. *When Your Child Has Been Molested: A Parent's Guide to Healing and Recovery.* Lexington: Lexington Books, 1988.
A practical guidebook. An essential companion for parents coping with the abuse of a child.

KRAIZER, CHERYLL KERNS. *The Safe Child Book.* P.O. Box GG, Palisades, NY 10964.
This is a clear, practical guide for teaching children skills to protect themselves. Reassuring, direct language.

SANFORD, LINDA. *The Silent Children: A Parent's Guide to the Prevention of Child Sexual Abuse.* New York: McGraw-Hill, 1980.
Detailed and practical. Resources for single parents, parents of children with disabilities, parents who are Asian, native American, black, and Hispanic.

Fiction & Autobiography

ANGELOU, MAYA. *I Know Why the Caged Bird Sings.* New York: Bantam, 1980.
A moving portrayal of incest and its effects in a wonderful autobiographical novel that celebrates life.

BARNES, LIZ. *hand me downs.* San Francisco: Spinsters/Aunt Lute, 1985.
A delightful autobiographical novel written from the point of view of a spunky five-year-old who is abused by her brother.

DICKSON, MARGARET. *Maddy's Song.* Boston: Houghton Mifflin, 1985.
A beautifully written novel about a young girl's struggle to break free from a physically abusive father.

FRASER, SYLVIA. *My Father's House: A Memoir of Incest and of Healing.* New York: Harper & Row, 1987.
Beautifully written, heart-wrenching, and healing.

LeGuin, Ursula. *A Wizard of Earthsea*. New York: Bantam, 1975.
Compelling fantasy about a young man's quest to seek out and conquer the shadows that chase him. Survivors of sexual abuse will have no trouble identifying with his denial, his search, and his recovery.

Morrison, Toni. *The Bluest Eye*. New York: Pocket Books, 1970.
A beautiful novel about a young survivor.

Murphy, Patricia. *Searching for Spring*. Naiad Press, 1987.
This excellent novel explores the healing of one member of an incest therapy group.

Swallow, Jean. *Leave a Light on for Me*. San Francisco: Spinsters/Aunt Lute, 1986.
An inspiring novel about a lesbian relationship between an incest survivor and a recovering alcoholic that actually works out in the end.

The Troops for Truddi Chase. *When Rabbit Howls*. New York: E. P. Dutton, 1987.
Written by the numerous personalities of a survivor of incest, this book shows how the mind must work to cope with the horror of sexual abuse.

Walker, Alice. *The Color Purple*. New York: Pocket Books, 1982.
A young woman's letters to God. Triumph through adversity. Exquisitely written.

Wassmo, Herbjorg. *The House with the Blind Glass Windows*. Translated by Roseann Lloyd and Allen Simpson. Seattle: Seal Press (3131 Western Ave., Suite 410, Seattle, WA 98121-1028), 1987.
This sensitive Norwegian novel shows both the vulnerability and the resilience of a young girl who is sexually abused by her stepfather.

Zahava, Irene. *Hear the Silence: Stories of Myth, Magic and Renewal.*
New York: Crossing Press, 1986.
Diverse crosscultural stories of women and spirituality. The first story
is a knockout about sexual abuse and retribution.

PERIODICALS AND NEWSLETTERS

For Crying Out Loud, c/o Women's Center, 46 Pleasant St., Cambridge,
MA 02139.
This fine quarterly newsletter is by and for women with a sexual abuse
history. A one-year subscription costs $10.00.

The Freedom Voice, published by PACA (People Allied for Child Advocacy), P.O. Box 17005, Durham, NC 27705, (919) 493-3333.
A quarterly newsletter published by this child rights organization
directed by victims and survivors of abuse. Champions the rights of
children and supports the recovery of survivors. "PACA is proud to
join the struggle of all people for equality, respect, and dignity." $6
per year.

Healing Journeys, P.O. Box 734, Centuck Station, NY 10710.
Healing Journeys is about healing together and sharing our strength
and experience to create a network of support, caring, and hope.
Members receive a newsletter, referrals, and other services. Membership fee is $35.00. Quarterly newsletter is only $9.95.

Incest Survivor Information Exchange, P.O. Box 3399, New Haven, CT
06515.
"Our purpose is to provide a forum for female and male survivors of
incest to publish their thoughts, writings and art work, and to exchange information." I.S.I.E. is financed primarily by donations, but
the newsletter will be sent to anyone who needs it at no charge.
Subscriptions are: $10.00 bulk mail, $12.00 first class. Sample issue:
$2.00.

The *"Looking Up" Times,* RFD #1, Box 2620, Mt. Vernon, ME 04352, (207) 293-2750.
   Looking Up not only produces this fine publication but also has excellent resources for Maine survivors of incest—therapy referrals, wilderness trips, art exhibits, training for therapists, legislative advocacy. Their mailing list is confidential.

The Newsy Letter, published by VOICES in Action, Inc., P.O. Box 148309, Chicago, IL 60614, (312) 327-1500.
   Available only as part of yearly membership in VOICES.

The Survivor Newsletter, published by P.L.E.A., P.O. Box 22, West Zia Road, Santa Fe, NM 87505.
   An excellent newsletter for male survivors. $20.00 for four issues. "We provide a communication network, share expertise, experience, and knowledge, and provide a mutual strength and support to adult male survivors."

Vermont-Incest Survivors Enlightened and Empowered (Vt.-I.S.E.E.), 24 Jonzetta Court, Milton, VT 05468.
   Includes information about books, conferences, workshops, & resources for survivors, as well as writing by survivors. Six issues cost $10.

ABOUT THE EDITORS

ELLEN BASS is a pioneer in the field of healing from child sexual abuse. Coauthor of *The Courage To Heal: A Guide for Women Survivors of Child Sexual Abuse,* she offers lectures and training for professionals nationally. She is also author of the children's book *I Like You To Make Jokes With Me, But I Don't Want You To Touch Me* and several volumes of poetry. She lives in Santa Cruz, California, with her partner, Janet, and their two children.

LOUISE THORNTON received her M.A. from the University of Illinois and teaches composition, creative writing, and literature at Gavilan College in Gilroy, California. She has written *My Brothers, My Sisters* and has co-edited *Touching Fire: Erotic Writings By Women.* She lives in Aptos, California, with her daughters.

JUDE BRISTER studied writing at the University of California at Santa Cruz, where she self-published two stories, "The Window's Netting" and "Tunafish." She lives in Vermont with her family, and cares for her daughter.

GRACE HAMMOND received her B.A. in women's literature from the University of California at Santa Cruz. She participated in training to develop the Child Assault Prevention Project, including the pre-school program, and developed and established CAP Projects in California. She continues to work on preventing violence against children and women by working with women's organizations and advocacy groups and by developing violence prevention and community-based programs. She provides proposal writing and program development consulting to non-profit organizations.

JEAN HUNTLEY (A.K.A. Rayjo) gives her highest attention to creating healing relationships—with her inner child, the people around her, and the earth. For many years she has given massage therapy with a physical/emotional/spiritual focus. She has come to see that individual healing is integral to an awareness of creating planetary healing.

VICKI LAMB studied in San Diego for her teaching credential in English, and worked on a psychiatric unit for children, most of whom had been sexually and/or physically abused. She lives in Fresno, California.